Handbook of Perinatal Infections

Quantity	Product Details
1	**Handbook of Perinatal Infections [Paperback] [1988] Sever, John L.** **SKU:** 2KG-18V-AFB **ASIN:** 0316781711 **Condition:** Used - Good **Order Item ID:** 164343822918641 **Condition note:** Cover has minor wear. Signature on first page. Five pages have a little highlighting. No tears or folds in text. Tight binding. Unused shipping charges on multiple purchases will be refunded back to you. Free tracking in the USA. Chris' Li'l Bookstore: selling new and used books since 2006.

Returning your item:

Go to "Your Account" on Amazon.com, click "Your Orders" and then click the "seller profile" link for this order to get information about the return and refund policies that apply.

Visit https://www.amazon.com/returns to print a return shipping label. Please have your order ID ready.

Thanks for buying on Amazon Marketplace. To provide feedback for the seller please visit www.amazon.com/feedback. To contact the seller, go to Your Orders in Your Account. Click the seller's name under the appropriate product. Then, in the "Further Information" section, click "Contact the Seller."

Thanks so much! - Chris

AP-TP - 1033648-1-0028
Main Address
800 Avondale Ave
1033648-1-0028
Grandview Heights, OH 43212

Buyer PO #: 1033648-1-0028

Order ID: 113-9910352-3217051

Thank you for buying from Chris' Li'l Bookstore on Amazon Marketplace.

Shipping Address:	Order Date:	Wed, Jul 8, 2026
AP-TP	Shipping Service:	Standard
Main Address	Buyer Name:	CollegeBooksDirect
800 Avondale Ave	Seller Name:	Chris' Li'l Bookstore
1033648-1-0028		
Grandview Heights, OH		
43212		

Handbook of Perinatal Infections

Second Edition

John L. Sever, M.D., Ph.D.
Professor and Chairman, Child Health and Development, Professor of Obstetrics and Gynecology, and Microbiology, George Washington University School of Medicine and Health Sciences; Senior Vice-President for Medical and Academic Affairs, Children's Hospital, National Medical Center, Washington, D.C.

John W. Larsen, Jr., M.D.
Professor of Obstetrics and Gynecology, and Genetics, George Washington University School of Medicine and Health Sciences; Director, Wilson Genetics Center, Department of Obstetrics and Gynecology, George Washington University Medical Center, Washington, D.C.

John H. Grossman III, M.D., Ph.D.
Professor of Obstetrics and Gynecology, and Microbiology, George Washington University School of Medicine and Health Sciences; Director, Division of Maternal-Fetal Medicine, Department of Obstetrics and Gynecology, George Washington University Medical Center, Washington, D.C.

Little, Brown and Company
Boston/Toronto

Second Edition

Library of Congress Catalog Card No. 88-82126

ISBN 0-316-78171-1

Printed in the United States of America

FF

Contents

Preface

The second edition of *Handbook of Perinatal Infections* provides completely updated information on topics of clinical importance for students, residents, and practitioners. There is new material on AIDS and parvoviruses as well as many changes in the material that appeared in the first edition. The concise format has been retained in order to facilitate quick reference. Each chapter has been organized to provide key information necessary for the diagnosis, management, and prevention of infection in the mother and child. Question-and-answer sections are included for those topics about which we have received frequent inquiries. Selected readings are provided at the end of each major chapter.

We are grateful for the assistance of Dr. Bishara Freij in the preparation of the chapters on neonatal sepsis and mycoplasmas.

J.L.S.
J.W.L.
J.H.G.

I

Viral Infections

Notice

The indications and dosages of all drugs in this book have been recommended in the medical literature and conform to the practices of the general medical community. The medications described do not necessarily have specific approval by the Food and Drug Administration for use in the diseases and dosages for which they are recommended. The package insert for each drug should be consulted for use and dosage as approved by the FDA. Because standards for usage change, it is advisable to keep abreast of revised recommendations, particularly those concerning new drugs.

1

Rubella

In 1941 Australian ophthalmologist Gregg reported seeing an increased number of children with cataracts following an epidemic of rubella in Sidney. Gregg recognized the association between maternal infection with rubella and this fetal damage. Shortly thereafter he identified the defects of the heart, deafness, and the other major findings of congenital rubella syndrome. More than 45 years later, investigators are still following the original children from Gregg's studies. In recent years, they have identified "late onset" defects, such as diabetes, in 20 percent of those followed.

FREQUENCY

Epidemics of rubella previously occurred about every seven years in the United States, although some rubella was seen every year, particularly in the spring. The last epidemic was in 1964 and resulted in more than 20,000 cases of congenital rubella. Since the introduction of the rubella vaccine in the late 1960s rubella has become quite rare, and only small outbreaks have occurred among certain unimmunized groups. Congenital rubella has almost disappeared, and only a few cases are now reported annually. The United States, Canada, and a few European countries routinely immunize all children. Japan, Australia, and England immunize prepubertal girls. The great majority of countries do not immunize for this disease.

DIAGNOSIS

Mother

Clinical

Diagnosis of maternal rubella is usually made on the basis of clinical findings and a history of exposure two to three weeks earlier (Table 1-1). Signs include a discrete pink-red maculopapular rash that begins on the face, spreads to the neck, arms, trunk, and legs, and lasts approximately three days. The rash may coalesce into a red blush, and an enanthem of red spots may be present. Lymph node enlargement, particularly of the suboccipital, postauricular, and cervical nodes is usually present. There may be a slight fever before and during the rash. Clinical findings are evident in approximately two-thirds of women who have rubella. The other third have inapparent infection. Confirmation of the clinical diagnosis requires serologic tests or virus isolation.

Serology

Antibody tests are readily available through private, hospital, or state laboratories and are now quite reliable. About 10 percent of women of childbearing age do not have antibody and are at risk for infection.

To document immunity, the patient should be tested for the presence of IgG-specific rubella antibody. This antibody appears at the time of clinical illness or about one month after immunization and persists for life (Fig. 1-1). The tests that are now most frequently used for IgG antibody are the hemagglutination inhibition (HI) test, latex

Table 1-1. Diagnosis of Rubella

Mother	Child (Congenital)
Clinical	
History: exposure 2–3 weeks earlier 3-day rash: pink-red maculopapules Begins on face and spreads to trunk and extremities. May coalesce to a red blush. Enanthem of small red spots Lymphadenopathy: suboccipital, postauricular, cervical Mild fever, headache, malaise, anorexia Conjunctivitis, cough, arthritis, arthralgia	Eyes: cataracts, glaucoma, microphthalmia, salt-and-pepper retinopathy Heart: peripheral pulmonic stenosis, patent ductus arteriosus, ventricular septal defect, myocarditis Head: microcephaly, encephalitis, mental retardation Deafness, thrombocytopenia with petechiae, hepatosplenomegaly, jaundice, microcephaly, mental retardation, pneumonitis, radiolucency of long bones Late Defects: diabetes, thyroid disease, and others
Laboratory	
Antibody seroconversion IgG (HI, latex agglutination, or ELISA) Specific rubella IgM antibody Virus isolation from throat	IgG antibody persistence more than 6 months (HI, latex agglutination, or ELISA) Specific rubella IgM antibody Virus isolation from throat, urine or spinal fluid

Fig. 1-1. Rubella antibody levels with various tests currently available.

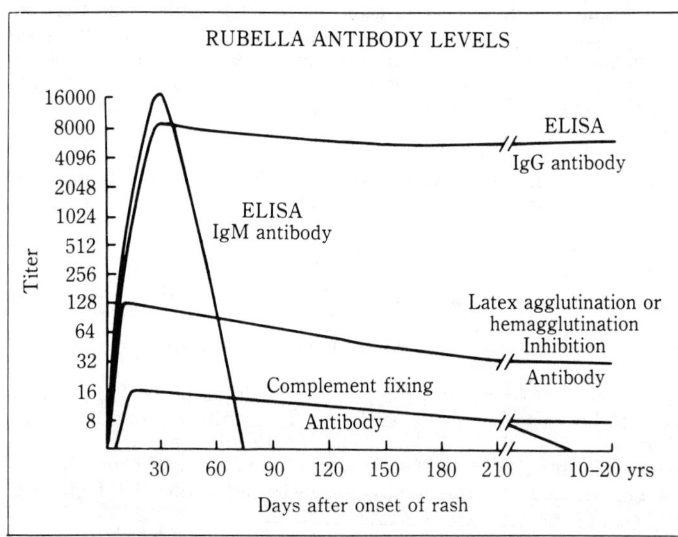

agglutination, or the enzyme-linked immunosorbent assay (ELISA) method.

To confirm a recent infection with rubella, the patient should be tested for IgM-specific rubella antibody. IgM antibody becomes detectable about one week after the onset of illness and persists for about one month. Thus, a single test can be used to confirm recent infection. In children with congenital rubella IgM-specific rubella antibody is present at birth and remains detectable for about six months. This is the test of choice for confirming the diagnosis of congenital rubella. Persistence of rubella-specific IgG antibody after six months of age but prior to immunization at 15 months can also assist in making a late diagnosis of congenital infection. The test most frequently used for IgM-specific rubella antibody is the ELISA method. It is important that the laboratory uses appropriate procedures to avoid false-positive IgM tests due to rheumatoid factor.

Antibody tests for IgG-specific antibody should also be used to identify women who are susceptible to infection. If no detectable IgG antibody is found, a woman should be considered at risk, and vaccine should be administered, provided she is not pregnant and will not become pregnant for three months after the vaccine is given.

Absent or low levels of IgG HI antibody are of concern because test results have been found to be in error in some laboratories. As with all tests, good quality control is essential. If there is reason to question the results, the sera should be sent to a reference laboratory and retested, preferably with one of the highly sensitive methods such as ELISA.

Virus Isolation

A second diagnostic approach is isolation of the virus at the time of the rash. The virus is present in the nasopharynx for approximately one week before and one week after appearance of the rash. Throat swab specimens should be obtained and sent to an appropriate virus diagnostic laboratory. Consultation concerning collection, storage, and transportation of the specimen can increase the yield of positive specimens. The clinician, however, should be aware that rubella isolation usually takes four to six weeks to complete and that this test is only available at a few laboratories in this country.

Child

Clinical

Classic congenital rubella can be diagnosed on the basis of the presence of cataracts, congenital heart disease (peripheral pulmonic stenosis, patent ductus arteriosus, ventricular septal defect, myocarditis), congenital glaucoma, radiolucent bone lesions, hepatosplenomegaly, petechiae, and thrombocytopenia. Some children have "salt-and-pepper" retinopathy, hearing loss, interstitial pneumonitis, jaundice, microcephaly, stenosis of various arteries, and, rarely, encephalitis. In most cases, however, the child with congenital infection exhibits only a few of these findings. The most frequent abnormalities are deafness and congenital heart disease.

Late-appearing defects have been found in children who have been followed longitudinally. These include primarily diabetes, which appears in approximately 20 percent of individuals at 10 to 20 years of age. Thyroid disease develops in 5 percent of patients and additional ocular damage in about 3 percent. In rare instances these children develop progressive rubella panencephalitis.

Serology

Laboratory confirmation of congenital rubella can be obtained by detecting IgM antibody in the child during the first 6 to 12 months of life. Elevated rubella antibody (IgG) persisting past the sixth month of life but prior to immunization is also confirmatory.

Daffos and associates (see Selected Readings) have reported antenatal diagnosis of rubella by ultrasound guided sampling of cord blood at 20 to 26 weeks' gestation. Rubella-specific IgM tests were performed on the sera. In one report 12 of 15 fetuses were found to have IgM-specific antibody. Parents were counseled that these 12 children had experienced in utero infection based on the findings. One of five children who did not have IgM antibody was found to have IgM-specific antibody at birth. Apparently the sampling was too early in that case. Clinical and laboratory follow-up data from this approach has not yet been reported.

Virus Isolation

Children with congenital rubella excrete virus from the nasopharynx for at least six months. Virus is also present in the urine and spinal fluid for a number of months. Thus, specimens for virus isolation may be used to establish the diagnosis, if appropriate laboratory facilities are available.

PROGNOSIS

Mother

The mother with rubella experiences only a mild disease that lasts an average of three days. In some cases, there may be mild arthralgia or arthritis of small joints and petechiae for a short period. Rarely, women have recurrent arthralgia or thrombocytopenia that lasts longer than a few days.

Child

Some newborns with severe pneumonitis and myocardial damage may die during the first weeks of life. For most children, however, the prognosis depends on the extent of permanent organ damage (Fig. 1-2). Significant permanent damage is found in approximately 50 percent of children with maternal rubella in the first month of pregnancy, 22 percent in the second month, 10 percent in the third month, and 6 percent in the fourth and fifth months. Some of the defects may become recognized only after prolonged observation. Thus, approximately one-third of defects in children with congenital rubella are missed in the newborn period because they do not become apparent until the children are several years old. The most frequent of these defects are deafness, mental retardation, heart and blood vessel defects, and diabetes. For this reason, repeated examination of children with congenital rubella should be conducted for six to eight years, to ensure early detection and treatment of major defects.

Severe late effects of chronic, suppressed rubella infection of the central nervous system are recognized as *progressive rubella panencephalitis*. In these cases, children with congenital rubella who were otherwise healthy through their second decade of life develop spasticity, ataxia, mental deterioration, and seizures. They have high serum and spinal fluid antibody titers to rubella and high spinal fluid gamma globulin levels. Rubella virus has been recovered from the brain of at least one child. This late disease is now recognized as one

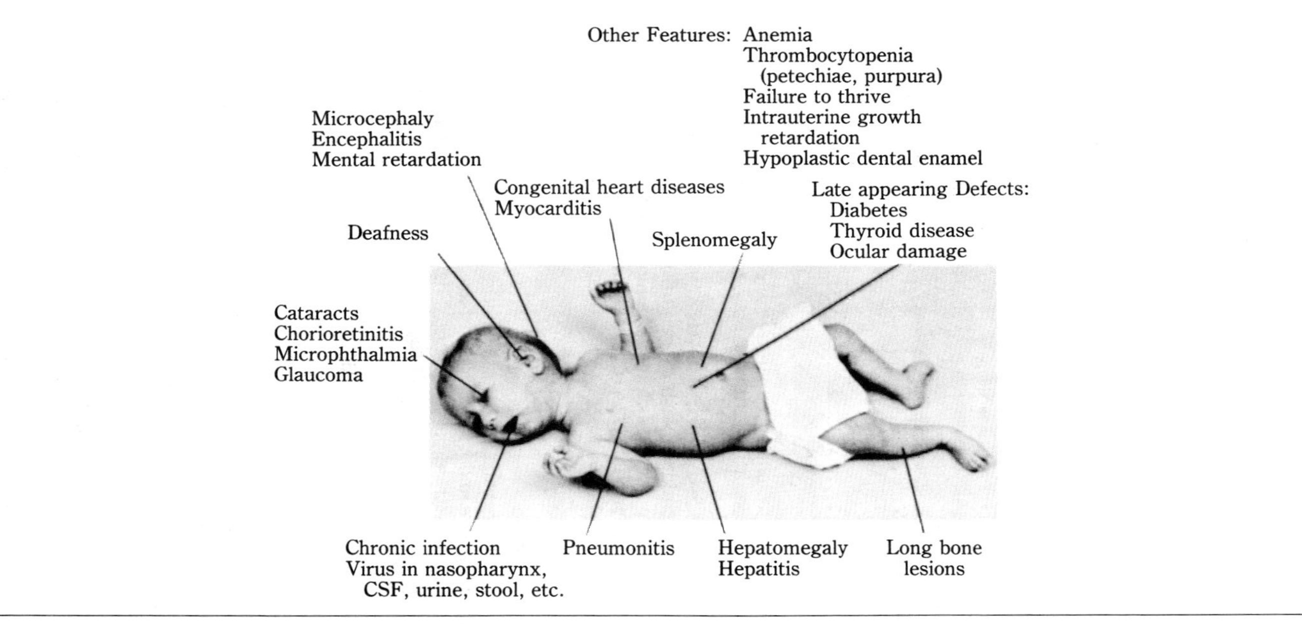

Fig. 1-2. Expanded congenital rubella syndrome. Clinical and laboratory findings.

Table 1-2. Management of Rubella

Mother	Child (Congenital)
Infection	
Mild analgesics Rest Document infection by serology or virus isolation	Isolate. Virus shed for 6–12 months Careful clinical studies for the type and extent of damage Repeated follow-up: clinical studies for defects and special treatment
Vaccines	
Immunize antibody negative women (10-15% of population have no antibody); make certain woman is not pregnant and will not become pregnant for 3 months Immediate post-partum immunization also useful	Immunize all children at 15 months of age and all unimmunized children before they enter school

of the manifestations of congenital rubella. The frequency with which this fatal encephalitis occurs has not been established, but it seems to be uncommon.

Additional late-appearing defects have now been recognized in over 20 percent of children with congenital rubella. Most of these defects appear at 10 to 20 years of age. The most frequent is diabetes (20%), followed by thyroid disease (5%), additional ocular damage (3%), and other defects (about 2%).

MANAGEMENT

Mother

Women with rubella require no special therapy (Table 1-2). Usually mild analgesics and a few days' rest are sufficient to control the fever, malaise, and arthralgia, if present. The physician's objective must be to document the occurrence of the infection by serology or virus isolation. If infection is established in early pregnancy, the woman may elect to have an abortion because of the increased risk of defects in the fetus. Patients with rubella should be seen at a time and place that minimizes the risk of spreading their infection to other susceptible contacts.

Child

The child with congenital rubella must be recognized as a potential source of rubella infection and should be isolated. Most children excrete the virus in the nasopharynx for about six months, but some children shed virus for more than one year. The child should be studied in detail to identify the type and the extent of the damage present. Defects of the heart and eyes should be treated by the appropriate subspecialists. Subtle damage, such as mild or moderate hearing loss and mild mental retardation, may not be established until many years later. Late-appearing defects such as diabetes may not appear until the child is 10 to 20 years old. For that reason, arrangements must be made for continued observation of the child and enrollment in appropriate special education programs as soon as possible. No antiviral chemotherapy is available.

PREVENTION

Vaccines for rubella have been available in the United States since 1969 and appear to be extremely effective. Approximately 95 percent of the people who are immunized develop detectable antibody, which persists for at least 10 years. "Mini" epidemics of rubella have occurred among small groups of unimmunized individuals, including college-age students and young adult office workers who did not receive the vaccine prior to 1969, religious groups that refuse immunization, and foreign students who are not immunized.

Physicians should recognize the importance of encouraging immunization against rubella. All children should be immunized. Current recommendations are that immunization be given at 15 months of age on a routine basis and that older children who have not been previously immunized receive the vaccine. In addition, women of childbearing age who do not have detectable IgG antibody should be immunized, provided they are not pregnant and will not become pregnant for at least three months after immunization.

The precaution against immunizing pregnant women is necessary because the present RA 27/3 vaccine virus has been shown to be transmitted to the products of conception in a few cases. Data from the Centers for Disease Control (CDC), however, have shown that among 153 pregnant, susceptible women who inadvertently received the RA 27/3 vaccine within three months of conception and who carried their pregnancies to term, none of their children had evidence of defects related to congenital rubella. Two of the children had IgM rubella antibody indicating that the vaccine virus infected the fetus in utero. Based on this data, if a woman accidentally receives the vaccine within three months of conception, the maximum theoretical risk for fetal damage is <2.5 percent.

Rubella vaccine may also be given in the immediate post-partum period. This approach takes advantage of the absence of pregnancy and the low probability that the woman will conceive within three months. Since pregnancies occur in some women immediately post partum (0.5-5%), appropriate precautions to avoid conception for three months are indicated.

In those special cases where Rh immune globulin is being administered for Rh incompatibility, rubella vaccine should still be administered, since the Rh immune globulin does not block effective immunization.

Several follow-up studies of immunization populations indicate that as many as 10 percent of vaccinated individuals have lost detectable antibody six to eight years after immunization. This probably indicates only a loss of HI antibody levels that can be detected with the current tests and not a loss of immunity. In the future, however, it may become necessary to repeat the immunization of those individuals who have lost all detectable antibody.

QUESTIONS AND ANSWERS

1. *IgM titer was reported to be positive 1:20. Does this indicate rubella?*

   No. That is the total IgM level in the serum. The test that is needed is for rubella-specific IgM.

2. *A pregnant patient traveled to Mexico and was probably exposed to rubella two weeks ago. She has no symptoms but wants to be checked for rubella. She was never tested for antibody and did not receive the vaccine. What test should be used?*

   Antibody to rubella develops 2 to 3 weeks after natural infection. If she has IgG antibody now it might be from a prior infection or it could be developing in response to this infection. An IgM rubella antibody test should be obtained about 4 weeks after the exposure. The presence of IgM antibody would be very strong evidence of current infection. A second IgG titer could also be obtained at 4 weeks. This titer should be greater than the present titer if this is a current infection.

3. *Rubella vaccine was given to a susceptible woman who was later found to have conceived about the time of the immunization. What is the risk to the child?*

   The CDC has followed 153 similar patients who have gone to term. None of the children had rubella defects. From this we can say that the statistical risk is <2.5 percent for a rubella-damaged child. Several children, however, had IgM antibody, indicating in utero infection. The vaccine virus has also been isolated from several products of infection. Thus, the vaccine virus is transmitted to the fetus in some cases. This indicates that with immunization there is a theoretical possibility for virus-related damage. For this reason, we do not recommend immunizing pregnant women.

SELECTED READINGS

Centers for Disease Control, U.S. Dept. H.H.S. Rubella Vaccination During Pregnancy—United States 1971–1985. *Morbidity and Mortality Weekly Report* 35(17):275–276, 1986.

Daffos, F. et al. Prenatal diagnosis of congenital rubella. *Lancet* (1):1–3, 1984.

Sever, J. Rubella vaccine given during pregnancy. *Perinatal Press* 8(1):3, 1984.

Sever, J. The menacing infections that spell TORCH. *Contemp. Obstet. Gynecol.* 25:109–123, 1985.

Sever, J. TORCH tests and what they mean. *Am. J. Obstet. Gynecol.* 152(5):495–498, 1985.

Sever, J. Rubella and congenital rubella. In R. Rakel (Ed.), *Conn's Current Therapy*, pp. 92–95. Philadelphia: Saunders, 1986.

2
Herpes

The number of physician office visits for genital herpes simplex virus (HSV) has increased rapidly in the last 20 years and is now estimated to be more than 300,000 per year. Genital herpes infections are generally due to herpes simplex virus, type 2 (HSV-2), while oral lesions are usually caused by herpes simplex virus, type 1 (HSV-1). Primary genital herpes infections with either type can cause severe genital lesions that frequently last for more than two weeks. Recurrences are usually less severe and last for about one week. Transmission of HSV to the child at delivery occurs in about half of pregnancies in which primary genital infection is present at term and the child is delivered vaginally. The risk is reduced when the delivery is by cesarean section or if recurrent HSV infection is present. Infections of the child may be very severe or fatal and can be caused by either HSV-1 or HSV-2, but are usually due to HSV-2 acquired by the baby at the time of delivery. Herpes infections early in pregnancy are associated with increased rates of abortions and, in rare instances, in utero infection of the fetus causing severe disease and damage.

The following definitions describe herpes infections and have been used by the World Health Organization (1985):

Primary infection	A first infection with any serotype of the virus (no prior antibody to HSV-1 or HSV-2)
First infection	The first infection of an individual with a given herpesvirus serotype, irrespective of an infection by other serotypes (no prior antibody to the serotype of the infecting HSV)
First clinical episode	The first clinically recognized disease; it may, but need not be, the primary infection
Secondary clinical episode	Any recognized disease episode occurring in individuals with previous clinical episode(s)
Latent infection (latency)	The presence in a particular tissue of the virus in a noninfectious form, which can be induced to replicate by specific stimuli, e.g., by the culture of tissue in vitro
Reactivation	The induction of replication of latent virus, which may, or may not, lead to clinical lesions
Asymptomatic shedding	Viral excretion in the absence of detectable clinical symptoms that may be the consequence of persistent virus multiplication or a reactivation of latent virus
Exogenous (super) infection	Infection of a previously infected individual with a virus of the same serotype from an exterior source; exogenous virus can be differentiated from reactivated virus only by laboratory techniques
Recurrent infection	Presence of virus at body surfaces or in secretions as a result of reactivation of latent virus, or as a consequence of reinfection with virus from an external source
Recurrent lesions	Lesions containing virus derived from reactivation within the dermatome or at or near the portal of entry of the virus into the body

Recurrent disease	Clinical manifestations that may follow virus replication in the host.

FREQUENCY

Studies of asymptomatic pregnant women in the general population have shown the frequency of positive cultures at the time of delivery to be 0.09 to 0.39 percent (Stagno and Whitley, 1985). The rates of infection among women attending sexually transmitted disease clinics have been in the range of 1.9 to 6.9 percent. In a study of pregnant women with a history of prior herpes, recurrent infections occurred in 84 percent of the patients, and the infections were asymptomatic in about 12 percent of the cases.

The frequency of neonatal herpes simplex is about 1:7500 deliveries (1:2500 to 1:10,000). In more than 60 percent of the cases the mothers reported no symptoms of HSV at the time of delivery.

DIAGNOSIS

Mother

Clinical

Primary genital infections are often quite severe and disabling but may be mild or asymptomatic (Table 2-1). Two to ten days following exposure, vesicles appear on the cervix, vagina, or external genital area. There is swelling and redness, and the external lesions may be quite painful. The only symptom of cervical lesions may be a vaginal discharge. Local lymphadenopathy is frequently present. The vesicles often open and become ulcerated (Fig. 2-1). The lesions usually persist one to three weeks, occasionally longer, and the virus is shed for a similar period. When reepithelialization occurs, virus shedding stops.

Following the primary infection, the virus travels up the sensory nerves and remains latent in the sensory ganglia. It may later become activated, travel down the same nerve branches, and produce recurrent lesions in the area of the original infection.

Recurrent genital infections occur within six months of the primary infection in about 50 percent of patients and then may reappear at irregular intervals. The lesions are usually few in number, smaller, and less painful than in the primary infection. Virus shedding generally persists for less than one week but may last as long as three weeks.

Herpes infection in pregnant women may, in rare instances, become disseminated on the skin or spread to produce hepatitis, thrombocytopenia, leukopenia, coagulopathy and encephalitis (Stagno and Whitley, 1985). Mortality with dissemination is approximately 50 percent. Treatment with acyclovir should be considered because of the severity of the infection; however, this drug has not been approved for use during pregnancy. If the drug is used, the case should be reported to the manufacturer (Burroughs Wellcome) for inclusion in its registry of pregnancy exposures. To date, acyclovir has not been shown to have an adverse effect on pregnancy outcome.

Virus Isolation

Detection of infection is best accomplished by virus isolation procedures with tissue cultures. Swab specimens are obtained from vesicles or ulcers by rubbing the base of the lesions. The specimens are taken to the laboratory in appropriate transport media at room temperature or +4° C. Specimens should be kept frozen with dry ice at −70° C if

Table 2-1. Diagnosis of Herpes Simplex Virus

Mother	Child
Clinical	
Herpetic lesions—cervix, vagina, genital area Vesicles become ulcerated and painful, persist 1–3 weeks Primary infection—multiple lesions, lymphadenopathy, no previous history Recurrent infection—few lesions, less painful	Localized (15%) Herpetic lesions on eyes, skin, or oral cavity CNS only (15%) Lethargy, anorexia, vomiting, fever, irritable. May also have localized lesions Disseminated (70%) Jaundice, purpura, respiratory distress, shock. May also have CNS and localized involvements
Laboratory	
Virus isolation—most sensitive Virus present 1–3 weeks Direct detection of virus Less sensitive (use only when virus isolation is not available) Smears of lesions (detect 60–90%) Specific fluorescent, peroxidase in situ hybridization and ELISA tests Pap smear for herpetic morphologic changes Serology Limited to retrospective diagnosis of primary infection. Paired sera or IgM-specific test. Some cross-reactions with other herpes viruses ELISA, neutralization, fluorescent and indirect hemagglutination (IHA) tests have some cross-reactions between HSV-1 and HSV-2 Most people have HSV-1 antibody and many have HSV-2 antibody	Virus isolation—most sensitive, from vesicle fluid, ulcerating lesions, nasopharynx, urine, and CSF Direct detection of virus Less sensitive, use only when virus isolation is not available Smears of lesions (detect 60–90%) Specific fluorescent peroxidase in situ hybridization and ELISA tests Pap smear for inclusions Serology Antibody in CSF and persisting serum titer strongly support the diagnosis IgM-specific antibody in blood in first 6 months makes diagnosis ELISA neutralization, fluorescent and IHA tests have some cross-reactions between HSV-1 and HSV-2

they cannot be tested in a few hours. The virus grows quite rapidly, and positive reports can be expected in one to two days, but may, on occasion, require up to a week.

A newer "shell vial" method reduces the time necessary for detection of HSV. The specimen is inoculated onto tissue culture that is growing on the bottom of a vial. The vial is centrifuged at low speed for a brief period of time (Gleaves et al., 1985). The centrifugation distorts the surface of the cells in the culture, and this increases the growth of the virus. HSV is then detected in the culture by specific fluorescence or enzyme-linked immunosorbent assay (ELISA) with labeled antibody (Michalski et al., 1986). This method provides a sensitive and specific 24- to 48-hour test.

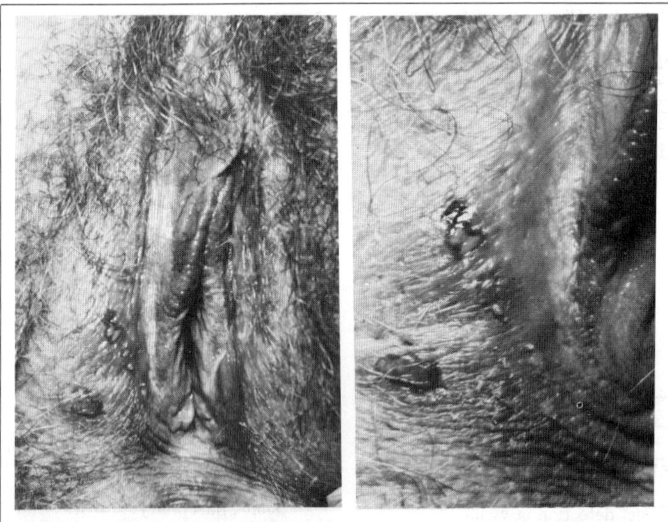

Fig. 2-1. Genital herpesvirus infection in the vesicular phase. Note vulvar edema.

Direct Detection of Virus

If virus isolation procedures are not available, several rapid, but less sensitive, methods for the direct detection of virus can be used. Smears of scrapings from lesions can be tested for HSV by using indirect fluorescence, peroxidase-labeled antibody or in situ hybridization tests. An ELISA antigen detection system with biotin avidin linkage is also available (Nerurkar and Namba, 1984). If these techniques are not available, Pap smears can be checked for the presence of multinucleation and inclusion-bearing cells (Fig. 2-2). These methods are more rapid than tissue culture but they will detect only about 60 to 90 percent of herpes infections.

Serology

Antibody tests are available but must be used with care. The majority of individuals acquire antibody to HSV-1 in childhood. In addition, HSV-2 infections begin to occur at puberty. In some populations, 30 to 60 percent of women of childbearing age have antibody to HSV-2. Because of cross-reactivity between HSV-1 and HSV-2 with almost all serologic tests, and the high frequency of antibody to these viruses, it is often difficult to confirm an infection on the basis of presence of antibody alone, particularly with the complement fixation (CF) test. Even the more sophisticated ELISA, microneutralization, fluorescent, and indirect hemagglutination (IHA) tests show some degree of crossing between HSV-1 and HSV-2.

The diagnosis of primary infection can be documented serologically by the demonstration of the development of herpes antibody using paired sera. Unfortunately, this change is often difficult to show because of serological cross-reactivity. The presence of specific IgM anti-

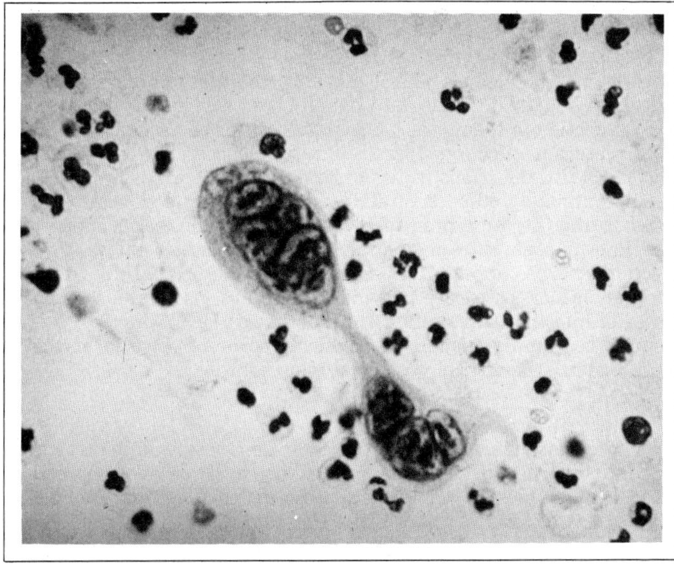

Fig. 2-2. Multinucleated giant cells suggestive of herpesvirus infection.

body to herpes for several months following primary infection can aid in making the diagnosis. Special techniques must be used to ensure the specificity of these tests.

Recurrent infections are common for both HSV-1 and HSV-2 even in the presence of type-specific antibody. Thus, the presence of antibody is not protective for recurrent maternal herpes or for neonatal herpes.

Child

Clinical

The great majority of perinatal herpesvirus infections are acquired at the time of vaginal delivery. An incubation period averaging 6 to 12 days follows before clinical symptoms begin to appear. The spectrum of findings may be divided into four main groups: (1) localized to the skin, eyes, or oral cavity; (2) nervous system alone or with localized infections; (3) dissemination to the visceral organs with or without involvement of the central nervous system (CNS); and (4) asymptomatic infections. About half of the infected babies are born prematurely. Skin lesions are seen in approximately half of the cases, and when present, they aid greatly in making the diagnosis.

Localized infection with herpetic lesions of the eyes, skin, or oral cavity occurs in about 15 percent of reported cases. Infection primarily involving the CNS with lethargy, anorexia, vomiting, fever, and irritability occurs in another 15 percent of cases. Disseminated infection takes place in 70 percent of reported cases and usually involves the liver and adrenals but may include the skin, CNS, and other organs. The first signs are often jaundice, purpura, respiratory distress, and shock. Asymptomatic infections are infrequent but have been documented.

Rare cases of in utero infections have been reported to result in severe fetal infection, neurologic abnormalities, or chorioretinitis (Hutto et al., 1987). These have usually been associated with primary HSV infection in the mother, but at least one case has followed recurrent maternal infection. Increased rates of abortion have also been reported with infections in the first trimester.

Approximately 90 percent of neonatal herpes infections are due to HSV-2, and the remaining to HSV-1. This finding is consistent with the known high rate of genital HSV-2 infections. A few cases of neonatal herpes appear to have been acquired postnatally from the mother, father, or a care provider. There are also well-documented cases of infection transmitted in the nursery. HSV-1 and HSV-2 appear to be equally capable of producing severe disease in newborns with a similar spectrum of clinical manifestations.

Virus Isolation

Specimens for virus study can be taken from vesicle fluid or ulcerating lesions. These lesions are most likely to be on the conjunctiva, nasopharynx, or skin. The swab specimens should be treated as described earlier (see Mother, Virus Isolation, p. 12). When no lesions are present, but the diagnosis is suspected clinically, or because of maternal genital infections, virus isolation should be attempted from the conjunctiva, nasopharynx, skin, and cerebrospinal fluid.

Indirect Detection of Virus

Whenever possible, children suspected of having herpes infections should be tested by virus isolation procedures at centers equipped to provide intensive care and treatment. At locations where special facilities and virus isolation tests are unavailable and when the child cannot be transferred, the specific and nonspecific staining tests of smears from lesions can be used (see Diagnosis, Mother, Direct Detection of Virus, p. 14). These tests are rapid but less sensitive than tissue culture methods and detect only 60 to 90 percent of infected lesions.

Serology

Virus isolation is preferred to serology for the diagnosis of herpesvirus infections. If viral culture techniques are not available, antibody tests can be performed using serum and spinal fluid. For these tests, the ELISA, microneutralization, fluorescent, or indirect hemagglutination tests are usually used. Each of these methods has some cross-reactivity between HSV-1 and HSV-2. A rising or persisting IgG-specific titer in the child over a period of six months confirms the diagnosis of infection. The presence of HSV antibody in the spinal fluid can also help establish the diagnosis. IgM herpes-specific tests can be used to identify antibody being made by the child in response to infection. Special methods must be used to separate virus-specific IgM antibody and to avoid false-positive reactions due to rheumatoid factor. Since antibody tests frequently do not become positive for a period of weeks to months they cannot be used for the early detection of infection.

Tests for viral antigen in the serum and cerebrospinal fluid (CSF) are under evaluation.

PROGNOSIS

Mother

The woman with primary genital herpes often experiences severe pain, burning, and itching in the area of the lesions for one to three weeks. In many cases, there is also burning on urination and swollen inguinal nodes. Frequently, a brief period of systemic symptoms, including fever, fatigue, and general malaise, is present. In rare cases, transient neuritis, urinary retention, meningitis, and death occur.

Recurrence of the genital infection may be asymptomatic, but, in many cases, lesions appear within six to eight months and then at irregular intervals—often several times each year for at least several years. The recurring lesions are less numerous, smaller than with primary infection, and may last one to two weeks.

Child

The risk of transmitting infection to the child during vaginal delivery is about 50 percent when the mother has primary genital HSV infection. With recurrent infection the risk is <8 percent (Prober et al., 1987; Brown et al., 1987).

Neonatal herpesvirus infection is often devastating to the child. Overall, 60 percent of the children die and about one-half of the survivors have significant permanent damage. More specific data for localized, CNS, and disseminated infections are as follows: When infection is localized to the skin, eyes, or mouth, as it is in 15 percent of the cases, the prognosis is relatively good. In one analysis of patients in this group, no deaths occurred, but permanent sequelae were found in about 30 percent of the children. If infection is localized primarily to the CNS (about 15 percent of children), then 40 percent of these children die; among the survivors, 70 percent have permanent damage. Disseminated infection, with or without CNS involvement, occurs in the remaining 70 percent of children. Among these infants, 80 percent die and half of the survivors have permanent damage.

MANAGEMENT

Mother

Chemotherapy to prevent or treat genital herpesvirus infections during pregnancy is needed but not available (Table 2-2). While acyclovir is helpful for genital herpes in nonpregnant women, insufficient experience concerning the perinatal consequences of treatment is available to justify routine use during pregnancy. Symptomatic treatment can be provided for the mother, including the use of Burow's solution topically, warm sitz baths, or warm dry heat from a hair dryer. Ointments and salves should be avoided, as they often spread the infection and retard healing. Various dyes, topical ether, cytosine arabinoside, 5-iodo-2′deoxyuridine (5-IDU), organic iodine, metronidazole, bacille Calmette Guérin (BCG), smallpox immunization, and other chemicals and potions have not been shown to be of benefit.

Delivery

The delivery should be accomplished in a manner that minimizes the exposure of the child to the virus-infected areas of the mother. Management requires the use of the best techniques available for detecting the presence of lesions or virus in the birth canal near term. When herpes is known to be present in the maternal cervix, vagina, or vulva, delivery should be by cesarean section.

Table 2-2. Management of Herpes Simplex Virus

Mother	Child
Maternal infection	**Perinatal exposure**
Specific treatment: none available for use during pregnancy Symptomatic treatment: Burow's solution topically Warm sitz baths Dry heat from hair dryer Delivery Primary infection at delivery gives greatest risk to child, but any clinical episode or asymptomatic shedding at term requires C-section Prior herpes with no lesions at term has low risk Delivery by C-section, preferably before rupture of membranes if lesions or virus are present in last week of gestation Postpartum Contact isolation and do not expose child until lesions are gone If mother will nurse, cover infected area and instruct on handwashing	Congenital (Transplacental) Maternal infection during pregnancy gives increased rates of abortion and rare in utero infection damage Abortion not recommended Neonatal Delivery by C-section, preferably before rupture of membranes Isolate, culture and observe carefully for 2–4 weeks. Specific treatment: Localized and CNS–use IV acyclovir Disseminated–Use IV vidarabine (See text for FDA restriction)
Prevention	
Instruct patient: Avoid partner with herpetic lesion. Use condom if partner has history of penile herpetic lesions. Avoid oral-genital sex if partner has oral lesion. Report signs or symptoms of herpes. Examine mother for clinical evidence of herpes. If prior history of herpes, culture near term. Deliver by C-section if evidence of herpes at or near term. If mother, father, or staff has oral herpes, instruct on handwashing and avoidance of kissing child and direct exposure.	Delivery by C-section reduces risk of infection.

Primary genital infection with herpes at term poses the greatest risk to the child. About 50 percent of children delivered vaginally to women with primary genital herpes will become infected. Delivery by cesarean section reduces this risk to about 7 percent. Every effort should be made to deliver the child by cesarean section prior to the rupture of the membranes. If amniorrhexis has occurred, cesarean delivery is still recommended regardless of the duration of membrane rupture, provided spontaneous delivery is not imminent at the time of diagnosis.

Recurrent infection of the mother at delivery has now been shown to have a relatively low rate of transmission to the child (<8%) (Prober et al., 1987; Brown et al., 1987). Since mother-to-baby transmission may still occur, however, patients with clinical evidence of recurrent infection at term should be delivered by cesarean section to further reduce the risk of infection to the child.

Patients with prior herpes and no lesions may have asymptomatic reactivation of infection at term. This is associated with a small but definite risk of transmitting infection to the child at delivery. This possibility has led to various recommendations for using serial cultures in the last weeks of pregnancy to attempt to identify asymptomatic infections at term. Unfortunately, no accurate five-minute "dipstick" test for herpes is available for use at delivery. The rapid tests that are available detect only 60 to 90 percent of infections and are least sensitive for asymptomatic infections, where only small amounts of virus are present. The most advanced, sensitive culture methods require at least 24 to 48 hours for completion.

A recent study of the serial culture approach has shown poor correlation between weekly cultures and the presence or absence of asymptomatic infections at delivery (Arvin et al., 1986). In 1987 this resulted in a change in the management recommended by the American College of Obstetricians and Gynecologists (ACOG): "It should be noted that there is no justification for cesarean delivery in women with a history of HSV infection but no active disease and in whom a culture is negative during the last weeks of pregnancy. Furthermore, cesarean delivery cannot be justified even when no culture has been taken and no active lesions are present" (ACOG, 1987). Based on this recommendation, then, women with prior herpes and no active lesions should be cultured at least once beginning at 34 weeks and, if negative, the delivery should be vaginal, even if no additional cultures are obtained. If the culture is positive, it should be repeated weekly and if negative within one week of delivery, vaginal delivery should be used.

Because of the poor predictive value of serial cultures for infection at term among asymptomatic women with prior herpes, it appears that serial cultures are of little or no value, and recommendations for cultures will be further modified or this practice will be discontinued. The resolution of this problem will only come when the accurate five-minute "dipstick" test for HSV is developed.

A pregnant woman with primary or recurrent herpes infection of the thighs or buttocks should be managed in the same manner as for genital herpes because infections in these areas are often associated with unrecognized genital herpes. If no clinical evidence of genital herpes is present in the last two weeks of gestation, the child may be delivered vaginally, but special precautions should be taken to protect the child from contact with the infected areas on the trunk or legs.

The infected woman should be instructed on the contagious nature of the herpetic lesions. If possible, she should undergo contact isolation procedures, and tests for herpesvirus should be made every two to four days until she is no longer infectious. If laboratory tests are not available, she should be isolated until the lesions have healed. If the woman wishes to breast feed her infant while still infected, the lesion should be covered, she should wash her hands, arms, and breasts thoroughly, and she should wear a gown.

Child

The child born to a woman with definite or probable herpes at term should be isolated and observed for the possible development of herpetic disease through 2 to 4 weeks of age. Cultures should be obtained from the conjunctiva, throat, and skin for virus at birth, and every two to three days. If clinical or laboratory evidence of herpes is present, chemotherapy should be started. The recent National Institutes of Health (NIH) Collaborative Study of treatment showed that if the herpes is localized to the skin or nervous system, intravenous acyclovir should be used. But if the infection is disseminated, intravenous vidarabine is indicated (Dr. R. J. Whitley, personal communication)*.

PREVENTION

Patients should be instructed on minimizing their exposure to herpes, including: (1) avoidance of genital contact when the male partner has penile lesions, and (2) the use of condoms when the partner has had penile herpes. The problem is complicated by spontaneous recurrences and asymptomatic infections.

The prevention of neonatal herpes infections must be directed at protecting the child from exposure to infected areas at the time of delivery. This protection is best accomplished by abdominal delivery prior to rupture of the membranes when virus or lesions are present (see Management, Delivery, p. 17). It is also usually recommended that the mother be isolated from the child until her lesions have cleared. The child should be isolated and checked frequently for evidence of herpesvirus infection and disease (see Management, Child). Breast feeding is permissible but precautions must be made to cover the infected areas and use handwashing to minimize exposure of the child to the infected area.

Women with active herpes lesions should be isolated in the hospital, and appropriate precautions should be taken at the time of cesarean section to prevent infection of hospital attendants and children. When the lesions have disappeared or the virus can no longer be isolated, the woman is considered noninfectious.

Since oral herpes can also be transmitted to the newborn, mothers, fathers, relatives, and staff with oral lesions should be instructed on handwashing, avoidance of kissing the child, and direct exposure to infected salivary secretions.

Vaccines for herpesviruses are under development.

QUESTIONS AND ANSWERS

1. *Can herpes be transmitted in utero when infection of the mother occurs in the first or second trimester?*

*Note: As of early 1988, intravenous acyclovir was not yet approved by the FDA for use in newborns. Vidarabine is approved for all forms of systemic herpes in newborns.

Yes. There have now been more than a dozen cases reported in which herpes early in pregnancy has resulted in in utero transmission and severe fetal disease. However, this is extremely rare, and abortion or treatment of the mother is not recommended.

2. *Should women with prior herpes be cultured routinely for herpes starting at 34 weeks' gestation?*

   "Official" recommendations on culturing asymptomatic women have been changing. In 1987 cultures were still recommended by ACOG, but if cultures were not obtained and the woman remained asymptomatic, vaginal delivery was advised. Weekly cultures provide very poor predictive information about herpes at delivery (ACOG, 1987). New, sensitive and specific rapid tests for herpes are needed for use at the time of delivery.

3. *What is the best laboratory method for detecting HSV?*

   At present the "shell vial" viral-culture technique is the best method for detecting HSV, since it provides excellent sensitivity and specificity and results are available in 24 to 48 hours (Gleaves et al., 1985; Michalski et al., 1986).

SELECTED READINGS

American College of Obstetricians and Gynecologists. ACOG Technical Bulletin Number 102 and Supplement. Washington, D.C.: March, 1987.

Arvin, A., et al. Failure of antepartum material cultures to predict the infants risk of exposure to herpes simplex virus at delivery. *N. Engl. J. Med.* 315:796–800, 1986.

Brown, Z., et al. Effects on infants of a first episode of genital herpes during pregnancy. *N. Engl. J. Med.* 317:1246–1251, 1987.

Gleaves, C., et al. Detection and serotyping of herpes simplex virus in MRC-5 cells by centrifugation and monoclonal antibodies 16h post-inoculation. *J. Clin. Microbiol.* 21:768–771, 1985.

Hutto, C., et al. Intrauterine herpes simplex virus infection. *J. Pediatr.* 110:97–101, 1987.

Michalski, F., et al. Enzyme-linked immunosorbent assay spin amplification technique for herpes simplex virus antigen detection. *J. Clin. Microbiol.* 24:310–311, 1986.

Nerurkar, L., and Namba, M. Rapid detection of herpes simplex virus in clinical specimens by use of a capture biotin-streptavidin enzyme linked immunosorbent assay. *J. Clin. Microbiol.* 20:109–114, 1984.

Prober, C., et al. Low risk of herpes simplex virus infections in neonates exposed to virus at the time of vaginal delivery to mothers with recurrent genital herpes simplex virus infection. *N. Engl. J. Med.* 316:240–244, 1987.

Stagno, S. and Whitley, R. Herpesvirus infections of pregnancy, Part II: Herpes simplex virus and varicella-zoster virus infections. *N. Eng. J. Med.* 313(21):1327–1330, 1985.

World Health Organization. Prevention and control of herpesvirus diseases. Bulletin 63: Part 1(2)185–201; Part 2(3)427–444, 1985.

AIDS

Acquired Immunodeficiency Syndrome (AIDS) was first recognized in the United States in 1981. The initial cases were primarily among homosexual and bisexual men, intravenous (IV) drug abusers, recipients of multiple blood transfusions, and individuals from Haiti. By 1983 it was clear that the sexual partners of individuals with AIDS were at risk for developing the disease and that pregnant women could transmit the infection to their children. The cause of AIDS was identified as a retrovirus by investigators in Paris (LAV virus) and at the National Institutes of Health in Bethesda, Maryland (HTLV-III virus). This virus is now called HIV (human immunodeficiency virus). AIDS has been reported to occur in almost all parts of the world. Studies in central Africa have demonstrated high frequencies of antibody to HIV and large numbers of patients with AIDS. HIV appears to have originated in Africa, probably as a mutant of a monkey retrovirus. A related but distinct virus, HIV-2, has been reported by some investigators to cause a similar disease in West Africa.

HIV has been isolated from blood, semen, vaginal secretions, milk, spinal fluid, saliva, and tears. Transmission has been shown to occur following exposure to infected blood or sexual contact. Children may also be infected in utero at delivery and by ingesting infected milk. One report has suggested possible infection by biting. No evidence of casual transmission exists (e.g., by sharing eating utensils, shaking hands). Accidental transmission to health care workers has been very infrequent and always related to direct inoculation or exposure of the skin to infected blood. One laboratory worker was infected while handling highly concentrated virus preparations. Transmission may have been by contact with the skin.

FREQUENCY

More than 50 percent of the cases of AIDS in the United States have been reported from New York City, Newark, Miami, San Francisco, and Los Angeles. By the year 1991, estimates show that there will be more than 270,000 cases; 9.7 percent (26,000) in women and 1.4 percent (3700) in children. In 1983 there were less than 100 cases of heterosexually transmitted AIDS but by 1986 there were over 1000 cases. Serologic surveys suggest that by 1986 more than 1 million people in the United States were infected.

Risk Groups

In the United States, AIDS in adults has occurred most frequently among homosexual and bisexual men (66%), homosexual IV drug users (8%), other IV drug users (16%), heterosexual contacts (4%), transfusion recipients, patients with hemophilia/coagulation disorders (3%), and infants born to infected mothers (1%). Of the heterosexual contacts, half were born in areas such as Haiti or central Africa, where heterosexual contact is thought to be a major route of HIV transmission. The remaining half were persons reported to have had sexual contact with a person who had AIDS or was at increased risk for AIDS. In this group, the majority were women (82%) and most had contact with an IV drug abuser (64%).

AIDS in children occurs primarily as a perinatal infection (78%). In the majority of these cases (73%), the mothers are either IV drug users or the sex partners of men who use IV drugs. Most of the children (70%) are from three states: New York, New Jersey, and Florida. This finding is consistent with the occurrence of adult AIDS cases in IV drug users, 75 percent of whom are from New York and New Jersey, and in Haitian immigrants, 79 percent of whom live in Florida or New York. It is expected that the proportion of children in other states will increase as the AIDS epidemic spreads to other parts of the United States. The other main risk group for children is made up of those who received blood or blood products between 1978 and 1985 (17%). With the availability of antibody tests for HIV and the screening of all blood for transfusions, the risk associated with transfusions has been almost eliminated.

Surveys of antibody to HIV in various populations in 1986 have shown the frequency of seropositive individuals to be the following: female blood donors—0.01 percent; female military recruits—0.06 percent; male recruits—0.15 percent; IV drug abusers—2 to 60 percent; female prostitutes—<2 to 70 percent; female partners of asymptomatic men with HIV antibody—10 percent; female partners of men with AIDS—47 to 71 percent; and Haitian women in the United States—4 to 8 percent.

Antibody Tests

Tests for IgG antibody to HIV are readily available. The enzyme-linked immunosorbent assay (ELISA) method is used first as a screening method. Positive tests are repeated, and if again positive a confirmatory test such as the Western Blot or the fluorescent method should be performed. Only confirmed positive tests should be reported to the patient, since false-positive results are more likely to occur with the screening ELISA method.

Tests for IgM antibody to HIV are being investigated but are not yet available for clinical use.

Virus Isolation

HIV can be isolated from blood and other tissues in research and specialized laboratories. This technique is generally not available in hospital laboratories. Tests for HIV antigen in blood specimens are being evaluated.

DIAGNOSIS

Mother

Clinical

The clinical course of AIDS in adults begins with exposure to HIV by blood or sex, followed by seroconversion, usually within 2 to 16 weeks. Many patients then experience infectious mononucleosis-like symptoms for a few weeks or transient signs of encephalitis. The patients are subsequently asymptomatic, seropositive and viremic for a period of months, years, and, in some cases, possibly indefinitely.

A proportion of HIV-infected patients develop AIDS. The most complete data is for homosexual and bisexual men. Many of these patients experienced repeated exposures to HIV and to a variety of other sexually transmitted infections. Based on this data, however, 10 to 20 percent were diagnosed as having AIDS within five years. By six years after infection, 15 to 25 percent of patients developed AIDS. The risk of developing AIDS in the same time periods may be somewhat

Table 3-1. Diagnosis of AIDS: Case Definition for AIDS for Surveillance Purposes*

I. Without Laboratory Evidence Regarding HIV Infection
If laboratory tests for HIV were not performed or gave inconclusive results (*See* Appendix 3-1) and the patient had no other cause of immunodeficiency listed in Section I.A below, then any disease listed in Section I.B indicates AIDS if it was diagnosed by a definitive method (*See* Appendix 3-2).
  A. Causes of immunodeficiency that disqualify diseases as indicators of AIDS in the absence of laboratory evidence for HIV infection
    1. High-dose or long-term systemic corticosteroid therapy or other immunosuppressive/cytotoxic therapy ≤3 months before the onset of the indicator disease.
    2. Any of the following diseases diagnosed ≤3 months after diagnosis of the indicator disease: Hodgkin's disease, non-Hodgkin's lymphoma (other than primary brain lymphoma), lymphocytic leukemia, multiple myeloma, any other cancer of lymphoreticular or histiocytic tissue, or angioimmunoblastic lymphadenopathy
    3. A genetic (congenital) immunodeficiency syndrome or an acquired immunodeficiency syndrome atypical of HIV infection, such as one involving hypogammaglobulinemia
  B. Indicator diseases diagnosed definitively (*See* Appendix 3-2)
    1. Candidiasis of the esophagus, trachea, bronchi, or lungs
    2. Cryptococcosis, extrapulmonary
    3. Cryptosporidiosis with diarrhea persisting >1 month
    4. Cytomegalovirus disease of an organ other than liver, spleen, or lymph nodes in a patient >1 month of age
    5. Herpes simplex virus infection causing a mucocutaneous ulcer that persists longer than 1 month; or bronchitis, pneumonitis, or esophagitis for any duration affecting a patient >1 month of age
    6. Kaposi's sarcoma affecting a patient <60 years of age
    7. Lymphoma of the brain (primary) affecting a patient <60 years of age
    8. Lymphoid interstitial pneumonia and/or pulmonary lymphoid hyperplasia (LIP/PLH complex) affecting a child <13 years of age
    9. *Mycobacterium avium* complex or *M. kansasii* disease, disseminated (at a site other than or in addition to lungs, skin, or cervical or hilar lymph nodes)
    10. *Pneumocystis carinii* pneumonia
    11. Progressive multifocal leukoencephalopathy
    12. Toxoplasmosis of the brain affecting a patient >1 month of age

II. With Laboratory Evidence for HIV Infection
Regardless of the presence of other causes of immunodeficiency (I.A), in the presence of laboratory evidence for HIV infection (*See* Appendix 3-1), any disease listed above (I.B) or below (II.A or II.B) indicates a diagnosis of AIDS.
  A. Indicator diseases diagnosed definitively (*See* Appendix 3-2)
    1. Bacterial infections, multiple or recurrent (any combination of at least two within a 2-year period), of the following types affecting a child <13 years of age:
       Septicemia, pneumonia, meningitis, bone or joint infection, or abscess of an internal organ or body cavity (excluding otitis media or superficial skin or mucosal abscesses), caused by *Haemophilus, Streptococcus* (including pneumococcus), or other pyogenic bacteria
    2. Coccidioidomycosis, disseminated (at a site other than or in addition to lungs or cervical or hilar lymph nodes)
    3. HIV encephalopathy (also called "HIV dementia," "AIDS dementia," or "subacute encephalitis due to HIV") (*See* Appendix 3-2 for description)
    4. Histoplasmosis, disseminated (at a site other than or in addition to lungs or cervical or hilar lymph nodes)
    5. Isosporiasis with diarrhea persisting >1 month
    6. Kaposi's sarcoma at any age

Table 3-1. (continued)

7. Lymphoma of the brain (primary) at any age
8. Other non-Hodgkin's lymphoma of B-cell or unknown immunologic phenotype and the following histologic types:
   a. Small noncleaved lymphoma (either Burkitt or non-Burkitt type)
   b. Immunoblastic sarcoma (equivalent to any of the following, although not necessarily all in combination: immunoblastic lymphoma, large-cell lymphoma, diffuse histiocytic lymphoma, diffuse undifferentiated lymphoma, or high-grade lymphoma)

   Note: Lymphomas are not included here if they are of T-cell immunologic phenotype or their histologic type is not described or is described as "lymphocytic," "lymphoblastic," "small cleaved," or "plasmacytoid lymphocytic"
9. Any mycobacterial disease caused by mycobacteria other than *M. tuberculosis*, disseminated (at a site other than or in addition to lungs, skin, or cervical or hilar lymph nodes)
10. Disease caused by *M. tuberculosis*, extrapulmonary (involving at least one site outside the lungs, regardless of whether there is concurrent pulmonary involvement)
11. *Salmonella* (nontyphoid) septicemia, recurrent
12. HIV wasting syndrome (emaciation, "slim disease") (*See* Appendix 3-2 for description)

B. Indicator diseases diagnosed presumptively (by a method other than those in Appendix 3-2)

Note: Given the seriousness of diseases indicative of AIDS, it is generally important to diagnose them definitively, especially when therapy that would be used may have serious side effects or when definitive diagnosis is needed for eligibility for antiretroviral therapy. Nonetheless, in some situations, a patient's condition will not permit the performance of definitive tests. In other situations, accepted clinical practice may be to diagnose presumptively based on the presence of characteristic clinical and laboratory abnormalities. Guidelines for presumptive diagnoses are suggested in Appendix 3-3.

1. Candidiasis of the esophagus
2. Cytomegalovirus retinitis with loss of vision
3. Kaposi's sarcoma
4. Lymphoid interstitial pneumonia and/or pulmonary lymphoid hyperplasia (LIP/PLH complex) affecting a child <13 years of age
5. Mycobacterial disease (acid-fast bacilli with species not identified by culture), disseminated (involving at least one site other than or in addition to lungs, skin, or cervical or hilar lymph nodes)
6. *Pneumocystis carinii* pneumonia
7. Toxoplasmosis of the brain affecting a patient >1 month of age

III. With Laboratory Evidence Against HIV Infection

With laboratory test results negative for HIV infection (*See* Appendix 3-1), a diagnosis of AIDS for surveillance purposes is ruled out *unless*:

A. All the other causes of immunodeficiency listed above in Section I.A are excluded; *and*

B. The patient has had either:

1. *Pneumocystis carinii* pneumonia diagnosed by a definitive method (*See* Appendix 3-2); *or*
2. a. Any of the other diseases indicative of AIDS listed above in Section I.B diagnosed by a definitive method (*See* Appendix 3-2); *and*

   b. A T-helper/inducer (CD4) lymphocyte count <400/mm^3.

Source: Centers for Disease Control, U.S. Dept. H.H.S. Revision of the CDC surveillance definition for acquired immunodeficiency syndrome. *Morbidity and Mortality Weekly Report* 36:1S–15S, 1987.

* For national reporting, a case of AIDS is defined as an illness characterized by one or more "indicator" diseases, depending on the status of laboratory evidence of HIV infection.

lower for patients in other risk groups such as individuals with hemophilia. Information for the long-term risk of HIV-infected individuals developing AIDS is limited since longitudinal observations were only begun in 1981.

The Centers for Disease Control (CDC) Case Definition for AIDS for Surveillance Purposes has been expanded and revised several times. The diagnostic criteria as of September 1, 1987, are given in Table 3–1 (CDC, 1987a). AIDS is diagnosed when patients experience one or more opportunistic infections or malignancies indicative of underlying cellular immune deficiency, with no known causes for the immunodeficiency. Patients with laboratory evidence of HIV infection (e.g., HIV antibody) are also included if they have HIV encephalopathy, HIV wasting syndrome, or a broad range of specific AIDS-indicative diseases. Patients are also included if the indicator diseases are diagnosed presumptively.

A CDC Classification System for patients with HIV infections has also been developed (Table 3–2). This system is based on the clinical findings that are present in the patient. The classifications are of greatest value for public health purposes such as disease reporting and surveillance. For descriptions of the classifications see CDC, 1986.

Serology

Almost all HIV-infected patients develop antibody that persists for life. An antibody test is an important part of the initial evaluation of all patients in risk groups and individuals with symptoms of AIDS. It is also recommended as a premarital test and for hospitalized patients. Some states have requirements for premarital tests; however, recent studies have suggested that premarital screening for HIV antibody may not be cost effective. In most cases, antibody does not appear in serum until 2 to 16 weeks after initial exposure. Thus, pregnant women in high-risk groups should be tested periodically during gestation to rule out the development of antibody during pregnancy. In addition, some patients lose detectable antibody in terminal stages of the illness.

Child

Clinical

The majority of children are infected in the perinatal period (78%). An infected pregnant woman has a 30 to 50 percent chance of transmitting the infection to her child. Most of the mothers are IV drug users (52%) or the sex partners of men who use IV drugs (21%). Similar high rates of drug abuse are found for all AIDS patients who are heterosexual. An additional 14 percent of the mothers come from countries where heterosexual transmission of AIDS is thought to be the major mode of transmission (Haiti and central Africa). A small proportion of the mothers have AIDS (3%) at the time of the pregnancy.

Most children with perinatal AIDS are from New York, New Jersey, and Florida (70%). The majority are black (54%) and the remainder are Hispanic (24%) or white (21%). Perinatal AIDS usually presents clinically by the age of 2 years (80%). Transplacental infection has been demonstrated, and several reports have been made of infection of infants by breast milk from mothers infected through transfusions given after delivery. Mothers are usually asymptomatic and undiagnosed at the time the infant is recognized as having the

Table 3-2. Classification Systems for HIV-Associated Virus Infections*

Mother

Group I Acute infection
Group II Asymptomatic infection[a]
Group III Persistent generalized lymphadenopathy[a]
Group IV Other disease
  Subgroup A Constitutional disease
  Subgroup B Neurologic disease
  Subgroup C Secondary infectious diseases
    Category C-1 Specified secondary infectious diseases listed in the CDC surveillance definition for AIDS[b]
    Category C-2 Other specified secondary infectious diseases
  Subgroup D Secondary cancers[b]
  Subgroup E Other conditions

Child

Class P-O Indeterminate infection
  Perinatally exposed infants and children up to 15 months of age who cannot be classified as definitely infected but who have antibody to HIV, indicating exposure to a mother who is infected
Class P-1 Asymptomatic infection
  Subclass A Normal immune function
  Subclass B Abnormal immune function
  Subclass C Not tested
Class P-2 Symptomatic Infection
  Subclass A Nonspecific findings
  Subclass B Progressive neurologic disease
  Subclass C Lymphoid interstitial pneumonitis
  Subclass D Secondary infectious diseases
    Category D-1 Opportunistic infections
    Category D-2 Bacterial infections (serious and recurrent)
    Category D-3 Other infectious diseases (oral candidiasis >2 months, herpes stomatitis-recurrent, herpes zoster-multidermatomal or disseminated
    Category E-1 Malignancies
    Category E-2 Other malignancies
  Subclass F Other Diseases
    Possibly due to HIV — e.g., hepatitis, cardiopathy, nephropathy, hematologic disorders (anemia, thrombocytopenia), and dermatologic diseases.

*For descriptions of the CDC classifications see CDC, 1986 and CDC, 1987b.
[a]Patients in Groups II and III may be subclassified on the basis of a laboratory evaluation
[b]Includes those patients whose clinical presentation fulfills the definition of AIDS used by CDC for national reporting

disease. Another group of children was infected by transfusion/blood products during the period of 1978–1985 (17%).

The most frequent clinical findings in infants with AIDS (90%) are poor growth, failure to thrive, chronic interstitial pneumonitis, and hepatosplenomegaly. Diffuse adenopathy occurs in about 50 percent of children. Less frequent findings include diarrhea, eczematoid rash, recurrent otitis media, developmental failure, and microcephaly. Lymphopenia is frequent in pediatric AIDS (20%) as is thrombocytopenia (40%). Radiologic evidence of interstitial pneumonitis is present in 90 percent of children with AIDS. Serum immunoglobulins are usually increased and T4 helper cells are reduced. Chronic lymphocytic interstitial pneumonitis is frequently seen in infant AIDS and has not been reported in adults.

AIDS is confirmed when a child has a reliably diagnosed disease at least moderately indicative of underlying cellular immunodeficiency but no known cause of underlying cellular immunodeficiency or other reduced resistence associated with that disease (Table 3–1). Congenital infections and hereditary immunodeficiency diseases must be excluded. A classification system for HIV infections in children has been developed (Table 3–2). For description of the classifications, see CDC, 1987b.

Serology

Tests for HIV antibody are almost always positive in pediatric AIDS. These tests, however, detect IgG antibody that crosses the placenta. Thus, the presence of HIV antibody in the newborn does not necessarily indicate infection of the child. Maternal antibody may be detected in the uninfected child for 6 to 12 months. In infected newborns, however, the HIV antibody generally persists and sometimes increases in titer. It is necessary to obtain serial antibody titers to demonstrate these patterns of antibody response. Tests for IgM-specific HIV antibody are under investigation.

PROGNOSIS

Mother

The long-term effect of pregnancy on the course of HIV disease is not known. Several studies have suggested that infected pregnant women progressed more rapidly from asymptomatic infection to clinical disease. A prospective study did not confirm these reports. Overall, 10 to 20 percent of HIV-infected adults develop AIDS within five years after infection, and 70 percent of patients with AIDS die within two years.

Child

Infants with perinatal HIV infection may develop AIDS within a few months after birth. About 50 percent are diagnosed as having AIDS by 9 months, 80 percent at 2 years, and 85 percent by 3 years of age. About 2 percent are not diagnosed until 6 to 8 years of age.

Half of the children with perinatal AIDS die within 11 months after diagnosis. Children diagnosed under 1 year of age have a more rapid course, and half die within 6 months after diagnosis.

MANAGEMENT

Mother

The management of pregnant women involves the identification of women in the following three categories: (1) those who are in a risk group; (2) those with acute infection (Classification Group I) or asymptomatic HIV infection (Group II); and (3) women with lymphadenopathy (Group III) or AIDS (Group IV) (Table 3–3).

Risk Group Only

IV drug abusers and sexual partners of IV drug abusers constitute the largest risk group (73%). Other important risk groups are women who come from countries where heterosexual transmission of AIDS is thought to be the major mode of transmission (14%) (e.g., Haiti and central Africa); women who are sexual partners of men with AIDS or who are at increased risk for AIDS; and women who received blood or blood products (1978–1985).

Women in these groups should be identified, tested for antibody for HIV (with counseling and consent), and examined for clinical evidence of HIV disease. If there is no antibody to HIV and no clinical findings, the women should be counseled concerning prevention of infection (see Prevention, p. 31). The antibody test for HIV should be repeated near term to identify women who may have become infected but were not yet seropositive at the time of the first determination.

Acute Infection (Group I) and Asymptomatic HIV Infection (Group II)

Women in this group come from the same risk groups listed above (see Risk Group Only). The presence of HIV antibody indicates that a woman has been infected and can transmit the infection to others, including her child. Such women should be studied carefully for possible early clinical or laboratory evidence of AIDS (see Tables 3–1 and 3–2). In some cases it is desirable to reconfirm the HIV antibody test.

These women should be counseled (see Prevention, Mother, p. 33). Clinical examinations should be repeated for possible development of AIDS. Psychiatric treatment, drug treatment, and support groups may be needed. Because of the instability of some families, child placement may have to be considered. Public education may be necessary to permit the patient to continue in employment, housing, school, and other activities.

Lymphadenopathy and AIDS (Groups III and IV)

Women with lymphadenopathy or AIDS should be counseled (see Prevention, Mother, p. 33). They should be observed and tested for possible extension of opportunistic infections, malignancies or neurologic abnormalities (dementia, peripheral neuropathy). These patients may benefit from psychiatric treatment, drug treatment, and support groups. Because of family instability and the illness of the mother, child placement may be needed. Public education may be necessary to permit the patient to continue in employment, housing, school, and other daily activities.

Women with AIDS may have opportunistic infections with TORCH agents such as cytomegalovirus, *Toxoplasma gondii*, and herpes. These infections require special consideration and management in relation to pregnancy (see Chap. 4, Cytomegalovirus; Chap. 22, Toxoplasmosis; Chap. 2, Herpes).

Child

Risk Group Only

Mothers who continue high-risk behavior should be advised to not breast feed because of the possibility of HIV infection and subsequent

Table 3-3. Management of HIV-Associated Virus Infections

Mother	Child
Risk Group Only	
Identify (primarily IV drug users or sexual partners of IV drug users) Test for antibody to HIV Examine for clinical evidence of HIV disease. If no laboratory evidence of antibody to HIV and no clinical evidence of infection— Counsel (See Prevention, Mother, p. 31) Repeat test for antibody to HIV near delivery	Do not breast feed if mother remains in a high-risk group
Acute Infection (Group I) and Asymptomatic Infection (Group II)	
Identify (primarily IV drug users or sexual partners of IV drugs users)* Examine for possible clinical or laboratory evidence of AIDS and test for antibody to HIV Counsel (See Prevention, Mother, p. 33) Repeat examinations for possible development of AIDS Possible need for psychiatric treatment, support groups, drug treatment, child placement Possible need for public education for employment, housing, school, and other activities	Child at risk for infection (30–50%) Do not breast feed Test for persisting antibody to HIV Examine for clinical or laboratory evidence of AIDS
Lymphadenopathy and AIDS (Groups III and IV)	
Counsel (See Prevention, Mother, p. 33) Observe and test for extension of opportunistic infections and/or malignancies Possible need for psychiatric treatment, support groups, drug treatment, child placement Possible need for public education for employment, housing, schools, and other activities Possible TORCH infections	Child at risk for infection (30–50%) Do not breast feed Test for persisting antibody to HIV Examine for clinical or laboratory evidence of AIDS Possible TORCH infections

*Most asymptomatic infected mothers who have a child with AIDS first become aware of their infection when their child is diagnosed.

transmission to the child. Also, if the mother was not tested for HIV antibody near term, the child should be tested to identify possible infection.

Acute Infection and Asymptomatic HIV Infection (Groups I and II)

Children born to mothers in this category have a 30 to 50 percent chance of being infected with HIV. They should not be breast fed because of the possibility of HIV transmission through the milk. HIV antibody titers should be performed in the newborn period and repeated every three months for one year to determine if there is a fall in titer, indicating no infection of the child, or a persisting or rising titer, indicating infection. The children should also be examined for clinical or laboratory evidence of AIDS (see Tables 3–1 and 3–2).

Lymphadenopathy and AIDS (Groups III and IV)

Children of women with lymphadenopathy or AIDS have the same risks for HIV infection and need the same management as that indicated above for children of mothers with acute infection and asymptomatic HIV infections. Additional considerations, however, are the specific opportunistic infections that the mother may have, such as cytomegalovirus, toxoplasmosis and herpes. These TORCH agents, if present, must be managed appropriately (see Chap. 4, Cytomegalovirus; Chap. 22, Toxoplasmosis; Chap. 2, Herpes).

PREVENTION

The prevention of infection of the child requires prevention of infection of the mother. Counseling of patients and education of the public is necessary to reduce the spread of HIV infections and to provide proper care and assistance for those who are infected (see Table 3–4).

Premarital tests for HIV antibody has been required in some states; however, required testing is considerably controversial. All U.S. military personnel are tested for antibody to HIV, and the testing of all prisoners and hospitalized patients is under consideration. All donated blood in the United States is tested prior to use.

Mother

Risk Group Only

These patients must first be identified by appropriate questioning. Since most are IV drug abusers or the sexual partners of IV drug users (73%), special efforts should be made to counsel and test these women for antibody to HIV. Additional groups of particular importance are women who come from countries where heterosexual transmission of AIDS is thought to be the major mode of transmission (e.g., Haiti and central Africa) and women who are sexual partners of men with AIDS or at increased risk of AIDS or have received blood or blood products (1978–1985).

Women in these risk groups who have no antibody to HIV should be counseled regarding the risk of becoming infected and methods to reduce that risk for themselves and their children. To reduce the risk, IV drug abusers should be asked to stop using drugs. If they persist in using drugs, they should be encouraged not to share needles and syringes and to enter drug treatment programs. Women should be informed about "safer" sex including the use of condoms and no exchange of body fluids (see CDC, 1985).

Table 3-4. Prevention of HIV Associated Virus Infections

Mother	Child
Risk Group Only	
Identify (primarily IV drug users or sexual partners of IV drug users) Test for antibody to HIV Examine for clinical evidence of AIDS If no antibody to HIV and no clinical or laboratory evidence of HIV infection: Counsel: Regarding risk for becoming infected Reduce risk by modification of use of IV drugs and/or sex practices Risk of transmission to child if infected (30–50%) Consider delaying future pregnancies Do not donate blood or organs Repeat test for antibody to HIV near delivery	Prevention of infection of the child requires prevention of infection of the mother Do not breast feed if mother continues in a high-risk group Test for antibody to HIV antibody if mother was not tested near term
Acute Infection and Asymptomatic Infection (Groups I and II)	
Identify (primarily IV drug users or sexual partners of IV drug users) Examine for clinical and laboratory evidence of AIDS Counsel: Regarding risk of developing AIDS Risk of transmission to child (30–50%) Risk of transmission to others by IV drug use (sharing needles and syringes) and sexual contact Refer drug and/or sex partners for counseling and testing Reduce risk of transmission of infection to others by modifying IV drug use and/or sex practices Do not donate blood or organs Inform physicians/dentists of positive antibody Consider delaying future pregnancies	Do not breast feed
Lymphadenopathy and AIDS (Groups III and IV)	
Monitor clinical and laboratory findings of AIDS. Treat as needed Counsel: Same as for Acute Infection and Asymptomatic Infection (Groups I and II, above).	Do not breast feed

Patients should be counseled that the risk of transmission of HIV from an infected mother to a child is approximately 30 to 50 percent. If they continue high-risk behavior, they should be encouraged to avoid pregnancy. These patients should not donate blood or organs. It is important to repeat the HIV antibody test near term to identify a seroconversion during pregnancy.

Acute Infection and Asymptomatic Infection (Groups I and II)

These women must be identified because of their symptoms of acute infection, including mononucleosis-like illness and encephalitis, or their risk behavior (see Risk Group Only). The presence of HIV antibody in these patients indicates that they have been infected and they carry the virus in their blood.

These patients are infected and must be counseled that they are at risk for developing AIDS and that they can transmit the infection to their child (30–50%). They can transmit the infection to others by blood-contaminated needles and syringes and by sexual contact. They should be encouraged to reduce the risk of transmission to others by discontinuing drug use. Minimally, they should modify their use of drugs (no shared needles or "works") or, preferably, should enter a drug treatment program. They should be encouraged to have safer sex (see Risk Group Only). They should not donate blood or organs. They should inform their physicians and dentists that they are infected so that appropriate precautions can be taken, and they should be counseled not to become pregnant.

Lymphadenopathy and AIDS (Groups III and IV)

Patients with lymphadenopathy or AIDS have HIV antibody and are infected. They have already progressed to the point of having symptoms of the HIV infection. They must be monitored for their clinical and laboratory findings and possible further development of opportunistic infections, malignancies, or neurologic abnormalities. These abnormalities can be serious, even life-threatening, and treatment must be instituted as rapidly as possible. Counseling for these patients should be the same as for the acute infection and asymptomatic infection category (Groups I and II) (see above).

Child

The prevention of perinatal infection requires prevention of infection of the mother. If the mother is in a risk group only she should be identified and counseled. If she has not been tested for HIV antibody near term, the child should be tested to detect possible infection. If the mother continues in a risk group, she should not breast feed because of the possibility of her becoming infected and transmitting the infection to her child.

Women who are infected, whether symptomatic or not, can transmit the infection to their child (30–50%) in utero, at delivery, or by breast milk after birth. Some women have had several successive infected children while others have had a noninfected child interspersed between infected children. Thus, all of these children must be studied for possible infection, and the mothers should be instructed not to breast feed.

QUESTIONS AND ANSWERS

1. *How is AIDS diagnosed?*

   The diagnosis of AIDS involves clinical and laboratory findings associated with immunodeficiency caused by HIV. The CDC Case Definition of AIDS For Surveillance Purposes (1987) is given in Table 3–1.

2. *What women are at greatest risk for infection?*

   Among pregnant women, the major risk groups are IV drug abusers or the sex partners of men who use IV drugs (73%); women from countries where heterosexual transmission of AIDS is thought to be the major mode of transmission (e.g., Haiti and central Africa) (14%); women who are sexual partners of men with AIDS or who are at increased risk for AIDS; and women who received blood or blood products (1978–1985). These women should be counseled and tested for antibody to HIV.

3. *Should cesarean section be used to reduce the risk of transmission of infection to the child?*

   Infection occurs in utero, at birth, and after birth (through milk). There is some preliminary evidence that cesarean section will not reduce the risk of fetal infection; however, more studies on method of delivery are needed.

4. *How can medical personnel reduce the risk of being infected?*

   HIV has been found in many body fluids and tissues. Precautions must be taken in handling fluids and tissues, particularly for self-inoculation with needles and exposure to the skin. Latex gloves should be used and gowns should be worn. If aerosols may develop, masks and eye protections should be worn. Mouth pipetting of specimens should *never* be used. Contaminated areas should be cleared with diluted bleach (0.5% sodium hypochlorite). The CDC has issued other recommendations for safety. (See CDC, 1987c).

SELECTED READINGS

Centers for Disease Control, U.S. Dept. H.H.S. Revision of the CDC surveillance case definition for acquired immunodeficiency syndrome. *Morbidity and Mortality Weekly Report* 36:1S–15S, 1987a.

Centers for Disease Control, U.S. Dept. H.H.S. CDC classification system for human T-lymphotropic virus type III/lymphadenopathy associated virus infections. *Morbidity and Mortality Weekly Report* 35:334–39, 1986.

Centers for Disease Control, U.S. Dept. H.H.S. CDC classification system for human immunodeficiency virus (HIV) infection in children under 13 years of age. *Morbidity and Mortality Weekly Report* 36:225–30, 235, 1987b.

Centers for Disease Control, U.S. Dept. H.H.S. CDC recommendations for assisting in the prevention of perinatal transmission of human T-lymphotropic virus type III/lymphadenopathy-associated virus and acquired immunodeficiency syndrome. *Morbidity and Mortality Weekly Report* 34:721–32, 1985.

Centers for Disease Control, U.S. Dept. H.H.S. CDC recommendations for prevention of HIV transmission in health-care settings. *Morbidity and Mortality Weekly Report* 36(Suppl. 2S) 1S–17S, 1987c.

Minkoff, H., et al. Pregnancies resulting in infants with acquired immunodeficiency syndrome or AIDS related complex. *Obstet. Gynecol.* 69:285–287, and 288–290, 1987.

Padian, N., et al. Male-to-Female transmission of human immunodeficiency virus. *J.A.M.A.* 258:788–790, 1987.

Parks, W. and Scott, G. An overview of pediatric AIDS: Approaches to diagnosis and outcome assessment: In Samuel Broder (Ed.), *AIDS: Modern concepts and therapeutic challenges*. New York: Marcel Dekker Inc., 1987.

Appendix 3-1. Laboratory Evidence For or Against HIV Infection

1. For infection
   When a patient has disease consistent with AIDS:
   a. A serum specimen from a patient ≥15 months of age, or from a child <15 months of age whose mother is not thought to have had HIV infection during the child's perinatal period, that is repeatedly reactive for HIV antibody by a screening test (e.g., enzyme-linked immunosorbent assay [ELISA]), as long as subsequent HIV-antibody tests (e.g., Western blot, immunofluorescence assay), if done, are positive; *or*
   b. A serum specimen from a child <15 months of age, whose mother is thought to have had HIV infection during the child's perinatal period, that is repeatedly reactive for HIV antibody by a screening test (e.g., ELISA), plus increased serum immunoglobulin levels and at least one of the following abnormal immunologic test results: reduced absolute lymphocyte count, depressed CD4 (T-helper) lymphocyte count, or decreased CD4/CD8 (helper/suppressor) ratio, as long as subsequent antibody tests (e.g., Western blot, immunofluorescence assay), if done, are positive; *or*
   c. A positive test for HIV serum antigen; *or*
   d. A positive HIV culture confirmed by both reverse transcriptase detection and a specific HIV-antigen test or in situ hybridization using a nucleic acid probe; *or*
   e. A positive result on any other highly specific test for HIV (e.g., nucleic acid probe of peripheral blood lymphocytes).
2. Against infection
   A nonreactive screening test for serum antibody to HIV (e.g., ELISA) without a reactive or positive result on any other test for HIV infection (e.g., antibody, antigen, culture), if done.
3. Inconclusive (neither for nor against infection)
   a. A repeatedly reactive screening test for serum antibody to HIV (e.g., ELISA) followed by a negative or inconclusive supplemental test (e.g., Western blot, immunofluorescence assay) without a positive HIV culture or serum antigen test, if done; *or*
   b. A serum specimen from a child <15 months of age, whose mother is thought to have had HIV infection during the child's perinatal period, that is repeatedly reactive for HIV antibody by a screening test, even if positive by a supplemental test, without additional evidence for immunodeficiency as described above (in 1.b) and without a positive HIV culture or serum antigen test, if done.

Source: Centers for Disease Control, U.S. Dept. H.H.S. Revision of the CDC surveillance definition for acquired immunodeficiency syndrome. *Morbidity and Mortality Weekly Report* 36:1s–15s, 1987.

Appendix 3-2. Definitive Diagnostic Methods for Diseases Indicative of AIDS

Diseases	Definitive Diagnostic Methods
Cryptosporidiosis Cytomegalovirus Isosporiasis Kaposi's sarcoma Lymphoma Lymphoid pneumonia or hyperplasia *Pneumocystis carinii* pneumonia Progressive multifocal leukoencephalopathy Toxoplasmosis	Microscopy (histology or cytology).
Candidiasis	Gross inspection by endoscopy or autopsy or by microscopy (histology or cytology) on a specimen obtained directly from the tissues affected (including scrapings from the mucosal surface), not from a culture.
Coccidioidomycosis Cryptococcosis Herpes simplex virus Histoplasmosis	Microscopy (histology or cytology), culture, or detection of antigen in a specimen obtained directly from the tissues affected or a fluid from those tissues.
Tuberculosis Other mycobacteriosis Salmonellosis Other bacterial infection	Culture.
HIV encephalopathy (dementia)*	Clinical findings of disabling cognitive or motor dysfunction interfering with occupation or activities of daily living, or loss of behavioral developmental milestones affecting a child, progressing over weeks to months, in the absence of a concurrent illness or condition other than HIV infection that could explain the findings. Methods to rule out such concurrent illnesses and conditions must include cerebrospinal fluid examination and either brain imaging (computed tomography or magnetic resonance) or autopsy.
HIV wasting syndrome*	Findings of profound involuntary weight loss $>10\%$ of baseline body weight plus either chronic diarrhea (at least two loose stools per day for ≥ 30 days) or chronic weakness and documented fever (for ≥ 30 days, intermittent or constant) in the absence of a concurrent illness or condition other than HIV infection that could explain the findings (e.g., cancer, tuberculosis, cryptosporidiosis, or other specific enteritis).

*For HIV encephalopathy and HIV wasting syndrome, the methods of diagnosis described here are not truly definitive, but are sufficiently rigorous for surveillance purposes.

Source: Centers for Disease Control, U.S. Dept. H.H.S. Revision of the CDC surveillance definition for acquired immunodeficiency syndrome. *Morbidity and Mortality Weekly Report* 36:1s–15s, 1987.

Appendix 3-3. Suggested Guidelines for Presumptive Diagnosis of Diseases Indicative of AIDS

Diseases	Presumptive Diagnostic Criteria
Candidiasis of esophagus	a. Recent onset of retrosternal pain on swallowing; *and* b. Oral candidiasis diagnosed by gross appearance of white patches or plaques on an erythematous base or by microscopic appearance of fungal mycelial filaments in an uncultured specimen scraped from the oral mucosa.
Cytomegalovirus retinitis	A characteristic appearance on serial ophthalmoscopic examinations (e.g., discrete patches of retinal whitening with distinct borders, spreading in a centrifugal manner, following blood vessels, progressing over several months, frequently associated with retinal vasculitis, hemorrhage, and necrosis). Resolution of active disease leaves retinal scarring and atrophy with retinal pigment epithelial mottling.
Mycobacteriosis	Microscopy of a specimen from stool or normally sterile body fluids or tissue from a site other than lungs, skin, or cervical or hilar lymph nodes, showing acid-fast bacilli of a species not identified by culture.
Kaposi's sarcoma	A characteristic gross appearance of an erythematous or violaceous plaque-like lesion on skin or mucous membrane. (**Note:** Presumptive diagnosis of Kaposi's sarcoma should not be made by clinicians who have seen few cases of it.)
Lymphoid interstitial pneumonia	Bilateral reticulonodular interstitial pulmonary infiltrates present on chest x-ray for ≥ 2 months with no pathogen identified and no response to antibiotic treatment.
Pneumocystis carinii pneumonia	a. A history of dyspnea on exertion or nonproductive cough of recent onset (within the past 3 months); *and* b. Chest x-ray evidence of diffuse bilateral interstitial infiltrates or gallium scan evidence of diffuse bilateral pulmonary disease; *and* c. Arterial blood gas analysis showing an arterial pO_2 of <70 mm Hg or a low respiratory diffusing capacity ($<80\%$ of predicted values) or an increase in the alveolar-arterial oxygen tension gradient; *and* d. No evidence of a bacterial pneumonia.
Toxoplasmosis of the brain	a. Recent onset of a focal neurologic abnormality consistent with intracranial disease or a reduced level of consciousness; *and* b. Brain imaging evidence of a lesion having a mass effect (on computed tomography or nuclear magnetic resonance) or the radiographic appearance of which is enhanced by injection of contrast medium; *and* c. Serum antibody to toxoplasmosis or successful response to therapy for toxoplasmosis.

Source: Centers for Disease Control, U.S. Dept. H.H.S. Revision of the CDC surveillance definition for acquired immunodeficiency syndrome. *Morbidity and Mortality Weekly Report* 36:1s–15s, 1987.

4 Cytomegalovirus

Human cytomegalovirus (CMV) was first grown in vitro in 1956. This permitted the development of laboratory techniques to define the frequency of the infection in pregnant women and the spectrum of clinical illness in children. Severe cytomegalic disease, which is apparent in the newborn period, is quite rare; however, more mild forms of damage that are not detected until later in childhood are much more frequent.

FREQUENCY

Primary infection with CMV occurs in approximately 1 to 2 percent of pregnant women. Previously infected women may also have recurrences during pregnancy. The virus can be isolated from about 3 percent of women at term. In sexually transmitted disease (STD) clinics as many as 15 percent of women are infected and excreting the virus. Virus shedding from the cervix, urine, or nasopharynx may persist for months to years. Congenital infection occurs in 1 to 2 percent of pregnancies. The risk of fetal infection is approximately equal for primary and recurrent maternal infections; however, almost all fetal damage is related to primary infection of the mother. While fetal infections can occur with recurrent CMV in the mother, fetal damage in these cases is very infrequent. Women in middle- or upper-income groups are more likely than women in low-income groups to be serosusceptible and experience primary infection; however, the risk of congenital infection is greater for women in low-income groups owing to a higher rate of recurrence of previous CMV infections.

If the mother is shedding CMV at parturition, the infection is frequently acquired by the child in the first months of life. By school age, 30 to 60 percent of children have antibody to CMV.

Some studies suggest that as many as 10 to 15 percent of congenitally infected children may have damage, primarily reduced hearing, related to this infection. Severe cytomegalic inclusion disease occurs in 1/10,000 to 1/20,000 newborns.

DIAGNOSIS

Mother

Clinical

Almost all maternal infections are asymptomatic (Table 4-1). Very rarely, infectious mononucleosis-like signs and symptoms may occur. In these cases, the heterophil test is negative.

Because the infection is almost always asymptomatic, studies of the association between maternal infection and fetal disease have required the use of laboratory tests to detect it.

Serology

Several antibody tests are available for CMV. The complement fixation (CF) method is no longer preferred because with this method, which employs frozen and thawed tissue culture antigen, there is considerable cross-reactivity with other herpesviruses and loss of antibody titer with time. Enzyme-linked immunosorbent assay (ELISA)

Table 4-1. Diagnosis of Cytomegalovirus

Mother	Child
Clinical	
Almost all asymptomatic Rare cases of mononucleosis-like illness	Severe (but rare) hepatosplenomegaly, thrombocytopenia, purpura, hepatomegaly, jaundice, chorioretinitis, pneumonia, pneumonitis, microphthalmia, microcephaly, hydrocephaly, hernia, deafness, mental retardation, cerebral calcifications Most frequent damage (10–15%) is reduced hearing
Laboratory	
Virus isolation best Cervical swabs, urine Serology Less sensitive Requires paired sera (tests often cross-reactive) IgM-specific antibody somewhat helpful (80–90% positive with primary infection, but 10% of patients with recurrent CMV also positive)	Virus isolation best Nasopharynx, conjunctiva, urine, spinal fluid Serology Less sensitive IgG antibody crosses placenta IgM-specific antibody helpful, if present

and fluorescent antibody (FA) tests are available through many laboratories. We prefer the ELISA method. Since 30 to 60 percent of adults have antibody, and since the finding of a positive test does not necessarily indicate recent or current infection, the use of serologic tests in clinical medicine should be restricted to symptomatic or high-risk patients who may have active or recent infection. (See Management, Mother, p. 41.)

In the rare case that a woman is suspected of having CMV infection because of mononucleosis-like symptoms, or for a woman that has been exposed to a patient with a CMV infection, the IgM-specific CMV test can be used to aid in diagnosing active or recent infection. If infection has occurred within the previous 30 to 60 days, ELISA or FA methods can show the presence of CMV-specific IgM. For these tests the laboratory must separate the IgM from IgG by ultracentrifugation or adsorption. These tests are positive in 75 to 80 percent of patients with primary infections; however, they are also positive in about 10 percent of women with recurrent infection.

Virus Isolation

The best way to establish the presence of CMV infection is by culturing the virus. Cervical cultures should be taken with a swab, placed in transport medium, and immediately taken to the laboratory for inoculation into human tissue culture. If a delay in inoculation cannot be avoided, the specimen, in transport media, can be held overnight at +4° C. Freezing the specimen or holding it longer than 16 hours can result in loss of virus titer. If specimens must be held or shipped, they should be packed in tightly closed containers that are kept cold with wet ice.

Using older methods, the detection of CMV from swabs or urine in tissue culture often required several weeks for completion. Newer methods using shell tissue culture vials, centrifugation, and monoclonal antibodies for FA give reliable results in a few days.

Child

Clinical

While approximately one to two percent of newborns are infected at birth, the great majority are completely asymptomatic. At the other end of the spectrum is the rare child with unequivocal cytomegalic inclusion disease. Most of these lesions (e.g., hepatosplenomegaly, thrombocytopenia, purpura, hepatomegaly, jaundice, chorioretinitis, and pneumonitis) result from damage that occurs relatively late in pregnancy. Other fetal damage includes microphthalmia, microcephaly, hydrocephaly, hernia, deafness, mental retardation, and, infrequently, cerebral calcifications. Fetal infection and damage is more likely when infection occurs in the first half of gestation.

Several groups of investigators have reported reduced hearing in 10 to 15 percent of congenitally infected children. To conduct these studies, large numbers of newborns are tested for CMV and then observed clinically for a number of years. Infection with CMV is also often acquired in the days or weeks after birth by contact of the uninfected newborn with the virus-positive mother. The infection can be transmitted from virus in the cervix, milk, pharynx, or urine of the mother or by blood transfusions from infected donors. This "late-acquired" infection of the newborn has been associated with pneumonia, hepatosplenomegaly and "septic" appearance in the first months of life.

Serology

While serology can be used to aid in the diagnosis of congenital CMV infection, virus isolation is more sensitive and direct. The CF test had been used for many years but ELISA and FA methods are more sensitive and specific. (See Diagnosis, Mother, Serology, p. 38.)

The great majority of children with congenital CMV have IgG antibody to this virus when tested with one of the newer methods. In the newborn period this can represent either maternal or fetal antibody, or both. In addition, about 70 percent of these children have IgM-specific antibody in the first months of life. Some false-positive tests also occur, and for the IgM test, the sera must be appropriately treated to eliminate cross-reactions, rheumatoid factor, and antibody complexes. The CMV-IgM, ELISA, or FA tests are available commercially.

Virus Isolation

The best method for documenting infection in the newborn is by virus isolation. Specimens should include the urine, nasopharynx, and conjunctiva. If neurologic symptoms develop, spinal fluid should be cultured.

PROGNOSIS

Mother

Acquired infection is almost always asymptomatic and without known sequelae. With the rare occurrence of infectious mononucleosis-like disease, moderate fatigue, malaise, fever, lymphadenopathy, and pharyngitis may be present for several weeks. Chronic cervicitis has also been reported in association with CMV infections.

Malignancies or intense immunosuppression may be accompanied by spread of CMV to the lungs, eyes, and other tissues.

Child

Primary infection with CMV during pregnancy is responsible for almost all cases of fetal damage. Women who have had previous infection with CMV can have recurrence of the infection during pregnancy and transmit the virus to the fetus, although these children rarely have evidence of abnormalities. The frequency of congenital infection due to primary infection in the mother is about equal to that associated with recurrent infection. Because fetal damage is almost exclusively associated with primary infection, the ability to distinguish primary infections from recurrences or persisting antibody due to previous infection would be desirable. Unfortunately, unless serum specimens are tested immediately before pregnancy and show no CMV antibody it is impossible to distinguish the forms of infection with complete certainty. Although CMV-IgM tests can be used, only about 80 to 90 percent of women develop CMV-IgM with primary infections and, at least 10 percent of women with recurrent infections have IgM. Also, the IgM may stay detectable for only a few weeks.

Estimates show that more than 3000 newborns are damaged by intrauterine infection with CMV each year in the United States. The permanent damage most frequently seen includes deafness and perhaps mental retardation. The more severe disease is quite rare and results in microphthalmia, microcephaly, hydrocephaly, chorioretinitis, and hernia. Since about 1 to 2 percent of all newborns are infected, it follows that about 90 percent of infected children have no clinical evidence of damage due to this virus.

CMV infection acquired in the first months of life has been associated with mild to moderate pneumonitis, which is self-limited. Most acquired infections are asymptomatic and there are no sequelae.

MANAGEMENT

Mother

The great majority of CMV infections are asymptomatic (Table 4-2). The rare case of infectious mononucleosis-like illness should be treated symptomatically and with rest. Immunosuppressed patients with severe CMV infections can be treated with antiviral drugs such as acyclovir.

Child

No satisfactory treatment is available, but several drugs are under study. Attempts have been made at using drugs such as adenine arabinoside, and acyclovir and related compounds for severely affected newborns. These drugs temporarily suppress the excretion of CMV, but virus shedding returns when the drugs are stopped.

Newborns who are symptomatic with congenital cytomegalic inclu-

Table 4-2. Management of Cytomegalovirus

Mother	Child (Congenital)
Symptoms	
Asymptomatic: no treatment needed or available Mononucleosis-like illness: symptomatic treatment and rest	Most asymptomatic and undetected Clinically ill: no satisfactory treatment available
Risk	
Primary or recurrent infection can result in fetal infection, but fetal damage is almost exclusively associated with primary infection	Isolate in hospital
Vaccines	
Being studied in nonpregnant populations	Would have to have been given to mother before conception

sion disease are shedding large quantities of virus, particularly in their urine, and should be placed on contact and respiratory isolation in the hospital. Personnel should wear gloves, masks, and gowns and use strict handwashing to minimize the exposure to seronegative pregnant hospital personnel and others who may be pregnant. (See Prevention, below.)

PREVENTION

Mother

CMV infection is transmitted by contact, the respiratory route, and venereally. Since it is usually asymptomatic, there is no easy way to detect the infection or to interrupt transmission. Chemotherapy is ineffective.

Some hospitals offer CMV antibody tests for women who work in delivery rooms and newborn nurseries. Individuals who do not have antibody and become pregnant are switched to other positions in the hospital during their pregnancies. For these purposes, care must be taken to use the more specific serologic tests such as ELISA. (See Diagnosis, Mother, Serology, p. 38.) Several studies, however, have shown no increase in the prevalence of CMV antibody or seroconversions among nurses working in "high-risk" areas such as renal transplant and neonatal units when compared to blood donors or other groups. These studies were not completely free of bias since special clinical and laboratory tests were being used in the higher risk areas to identify infected patients, and nurses caring for these patients were usually instructed to wear gowns and gloves and were required to wash their hands. Thus, the risk of transmission of CMV may have been greater in the study areas but reduced by the special precautions that were being employed.

Studies with attenuated CMV vaccines are in progress on both normal volunteers and selected patients who are to undergo renal transplants. Concern exists about possible hazards related to the parenteral administration of CMV since this virus is known to produce chronic infection.

Child

The prevention of congenital infection must depend on prevention of infection of the mother, presumably by the development of safe, effective vaccines. With natural infections, however, it is now recognized that several children can be born congenitally infected from the same mother. This suggests that, in a similar way, the vaccine virus itself might become latent or chronic in an immunized woman, only to be transmitted to her children in subsequent pregnancies. Obviously, it will be important to establish the safety of the vaccine, not only for the immunized woman but also for her children born in later years.

QUESTIONS AND ANSWERS

1. *Should all women be tested for CMV antibody during pregnancy?*

   We do not recommend routine testing. For routine testing to be effective, women would have to be tested before becoming pregnant and, if negative, tested again later in pregnancy. About 2 percent would be expected to seroconvert from negative to positive during pregnancy. No treatment is available, and counseling for possible therapeutic abortion would be necessary. The risk of fetal infection is about 50 percent, and among the infected children approximately 10 to 15 percent would be expected to have some later evidence of damage—mostly limited to reduced hearing. Among 1000 pregnant women, then, one might expect to have one child with reduced hearing due to CMV; however, as many as 20 unnecessary therapeutic abortions might be performed on the basis of the serologic tests. In addition, 300 to 600 women would have preexisting CMV antibody due to prior infections and, if prepregnancy sera were not available, CMV-IgM tests would have to be used to attempt to distinguish these women from the 20 with primary infections. If tests are used they should be limited to high-risk women and the ELISA method should be used. The IgM tests are of limited value since only 70 percent of women with the primary infections develop CMV-IgM antibody, and 10 percent of women with recurrent infections also have positive CMV-IgM tests.

2. *Is the risk of fetal infection and damage different for primary versus recurrent CMV in the mother?*

   Yes. The overall frequency of congenital infection in newborns is approximately equal as a result of primary or recurrent maternal CMV infections—each about 0.5–2 percent. Actually, the rate of congenital infection with primary infection is much higher (50%) than the risk for fetal infection among previously seropositive women (1%); however, only about 2 percent of women experience primary infection during pregnancy, and this influences the total number of children that are infected. Fetal damage is almost exclusively associated with primary infection in the mother.

SELECTED READINGS

Bale, J., et al. Congenital cytomegalovirus infection. *Am. J. Dis. Child.* 140:128–131, 1986.

Balfour, C., and Balfour, H. Cytomegalovirus is not an occupational risk for nurses in renal transplant and neonatal units: Results of a prospective study. *J.A.M.A.* 256:1909–1914, 1986.

Chandler, S., Alexander, E. and Holmes, K. Epidemiology of cytomegaloviral infection in a heterogeneous population of pregnant women. *J. Infect. Dis.* 152:249–256, 1985.

Handsfield, H., et al. Cytomegalovirus infection in sex partners: Evidence for sexual transmission. *J. Infect. Dis.* 151:344–348, 1985.

Stagno, S., et al. Congenital cytomegalovirus infection—the relative importance of primary and recurrent maternal infection. *N. Engl. J. Med.* 306:945–949, 1982.

Stagno, S., et al. Immunoglobulin M antibodies detected by enzyme-linked immunosorbent assay and radioimunoassay in the diagnosis of cytomegalovirus infections in pregnant women and newborn infants. *J. Clin. Microbiol.* 21:930–935, 1985.

Stagno, S., et al. Primary cytomegalovirus infection in pregnancy—incidence, transmission to fetus, and clinical outcome. *J.A.M.A.* 256: 1904–1908, 1986.

5

Varicella-Zoster

Infants with congenital varicella-zoster (chickenpox-shingles) have a variety of defects including skin scarring, muscle atrophy, hypoplastic extremities, chorioretinitis, encephalitis, and cortical atrophy. The damage appears to be due to the development of herpes zoster-like disease in utero and an associated encephalitis. Most malformations occur with maternal varicella in the first 20 weeks of gestation. When infection occurs later in gestation the child may experience zoster a few months to several years after birth. Maternal varicella 5 to 21 days before term can be transmitted in utero, and the child may have mild chickenpox at birth or in the first few days of life.

In addition to the fetal malformations associated with varicella in pregnancy, maternal chickenpox appearing the last five days of gestation or up to 48 hours after delivery can result in severe, sometimes fatal, generalized infection of the newborn.

FREQUENCY

Varicella is relatively infrequent during pregnancy. In the Collaborative Perinatal Research Study, eight cases in 60,000 pregnancies (1/7500) were reported (see Sever reference in Selected Readings). All of the infections were in the second or third trimester of pregnancy and none of the children had evidence of congenital disease.

Congenital varicella was not recognized before 1947. Since the reporting of cases has been far from complete, the degree of risk to the fetus due to maternal varicella cannot be accurately estimated. The frequency of damage, however, is probably less than 3 percent, and almost all defects are associated with maternal varicella at ≤ 20 weeks gestation. There is one report of fetal damage when the mother had varicella at 28 weeks' gestation.

The same virus that produces varicella (chickenpox) on primary infection may remain latent in the nerve roots for many years. In some individuals, it becomes activated and travels down the nerve to produce zoster (shingles). Maternal zoster has been suggested as a cause of some congenital defects. These cases are poorly documented and may represent atypical maternal varicella or other infections. There is one case, however, of typical congenital varicella associated with maternal herpes zoster varicellosus.

DIAGNOSIS

Mother

Clinical

Varicella is highly contagious (Table 5-1). The incubation period is 10 to 20 days, and the disease begins with fever, malaise, and rash. The rash is characteristic and comes out in crops on the trunk (Fig. 5-1) and, to a lesser extent, on the face, scalp, and extremities. Each lesion progresses rapidly from a macule to a papule to a vesicle that crusts over (Fig. 5-2). New lesions generally appear for three to five days and scabs appear for another three to four days. Characteristically, lesions in all stages can be seen in the same general area.

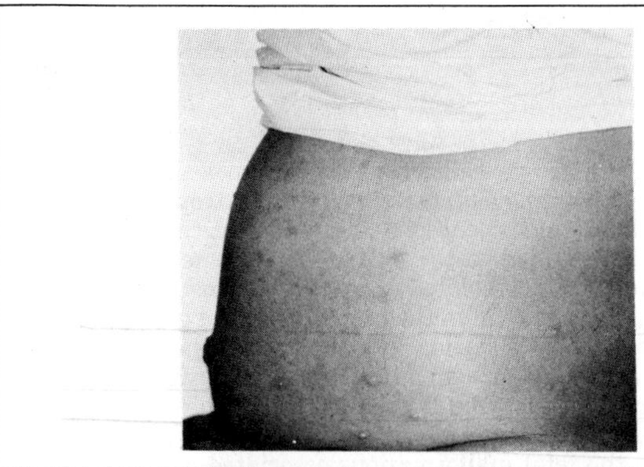

Fig. 5-1. Varicella rash during the third trimester of pregnancy.

Table 5-1. Diagnosis of Varicella

Mother	Child
Clinical	
History of exposure Incubation 10–20 days Fever, malaise Rash in crops Macule, papule, vesicle Lesions in various stages Mainly on trunk, less on face, arms and legs	Early congenital infection Low birth weight Motor-sensory paralysis Failure to thrive Skin scarring Muscle atrophy Hypoplastic extremity Atrophic digits Chorioretinitis Microphthalmia Nystagmus Club feet Encephalitis Cortical atrophy Repeated infection Infantile zoster Late congenital infection (last 3 weeks) Maternal infection: last 5 days to 48 hours after delivery results in severe disseminated neonatal infection (30% die) Maternal varicella: 5–21 days before delivery can result in mild chickenpox in newborn
Laboratory	
Virus isolation Direct inoculation into tissue culture Viral antigen from vesicular fluid by gel or CIE tests. Serology ELISA, FAMA	Congenital infection Virus not recovered Use ELISA or FAMA IgM-specific tests. After 6 months IgG-ELISA or FAMA since antibody persists. Late congenital infection Same tests as for acquired infection in mother

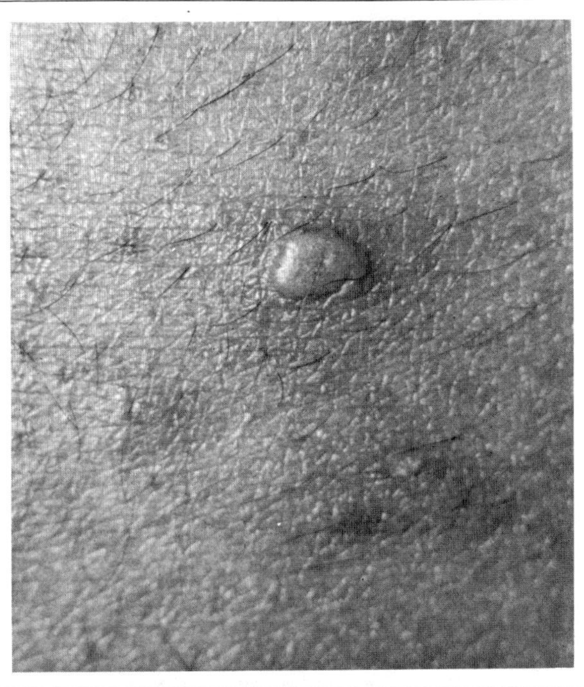

Fig. 5-2. A typical varicella vesicle. Note adjacent macules that subsequently become vesicles.

Virus Isolation

Varicella virus can be isolated from vesicular fluid the first four days of rash. The fluid should be inoculated directly into human fetal fibroblast cultures. Viral antigen can also be demonstrated in vesicular fluid by gel diffusion tests or counter immunoelectrophoresis (CIE).

Serology

To determine if a woman is immune or susceptible, the tests of choice are enzyme-linked immunosorbent assay (ELISA) or fluorescent antibody membrane antigen (FAMA) for IgG antibody to varicella. ELISA tests are available through larger commercial laboratories.

Child: Early Congenital Infection

Clinical

The child with congenital damage due to maternal infection during the first five months of pregnancy may have a variety of abnormalities, including low birth weight, motor-sensory paralysis, failure to thrive, skin scarring with muscle atrophy, hypoplastic extremity, atrophic digits, chorioretinitis, and other defects (Fig. 5-3). Some of these children also have zoster during infancy. In addition, some chil-

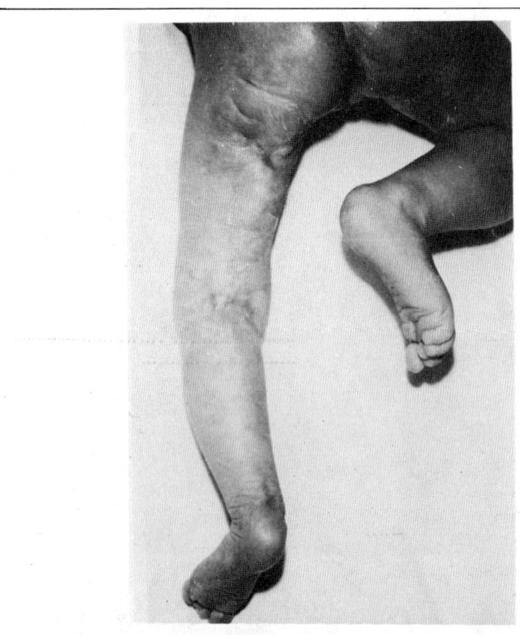

Fig. 5-3. Congenital varicella with skin scarring, muscle atrophy, and hypoplastic extremity. The child also had cortical atrophy and mental retardation.

dren born to women who have varicella in the last four months of gestation may have zoster during the first one to five years of life.

Laboratory

Virus has not been recovered from these infants. The IgG antibody to varicella, which persists over a period of years, can be used to assist in making the diagnosis. We prefer to use the ELISA or FAMA tests. IgM-specific antibody to varicella has been found in some of the infants studied in the first months of life. This test requires adsorption of the serum prior to testing with the ELISA or FAMA method.

Child: Late Congenital Infection (Last Three Weeks)

Clinical

Maternal varicella in the last five days of gestation or within 48 hours after delivery can be transmitted by viremic spread to the child. About 30 percent of such children die of disseminated infection. Varicella lesions appear five to ten days after birth and develop over a period of several days. The rash is often very extensive and pneumonia occurs, which may lead to death. Autopsy studies show widespread dissemination of the infection.

Maternal varicella five days to three weeks before term can also result in varicella of the newborn. Typical lesions develop on the skin of the child within the first four days of life. The disease is generally mild.

Table 5-2. Management of Varicella

Mother	Child
Following Exposure: Test for IgG antibody with ELISA or FAMA 95% are immune If negative, can give VZIG within 72 hrs of exposure This may reduce severity of infection For Varicella-Zoster: Symptomatic treatment Rare complications Bacterial infection of lesions Encephalitis Varicella pneumonia Isolate if in hospital Use contact isolation Respiratory isolation if varicella pneumonia For Severe Illness: Consider possible treatment with vidarabine or acyclovir	Early congenital infection Treat congenital defects No isolation necessary, not infectious Late congenital infection (last 3 weeks) Maternal infection last 5 days to 48 hours after delivery; give VZIG to child within 72 hours after birth Isolate child if varicella develops Maternal varicella 5–21 days before delivery Treat varicella in child symptomatically Isolate if in hospital

Laboratory

Virus isolation, viral antigens, and serologic tests are the same as those used for acquired infection in the mother. (See Diagnosis, Mother, Virus Isolation, Serology, p. 47.)

MANAGEMENT

Mother

Treatment is symptomatic (Table 5-2). Acetaminophen should be used for fever, and calamine lotion or similar topical applications for itching. Infrequent to rare complications include bacterial infection of the lesions, encephalitis, and varicella pneumonia.

Adults with varicella frequently experience illness more severe than that seen in children. Overall, pneumonia occurs in 14 percent of adults, and 3 percent die. For life-threatening illness, treatment with ventilatory support and vidarabine or acyclovir may be lifesaving. These drugs, however, are not approved for this use, and data on possible fetal damage due to the drugs are very limited. Vidarabine is teratogenic in laboratory animals, while acyclovir is not.

Child

Varicella-Zoster immune globulin (VZIG) is available through the American Red Cross Regional Centers for newborns when the mother has experienced varicella in the last five days of her pregnancy or within 48 hours after delivery. This should be given to the child to prevent or modify the infection. It must be administered within 72 hours of birth. This approach is not always effective since there is at least one report of neonatal infection with damage after the appropriate use of VZIG.

PREVENTION

Mother

Since varicella is extremely communicable, mothers or newborns with clinical chickenpox should be isolated. Infection is spread by direct and indirect contact and by the respiratory route. Isolation should be for contact and respiratory transmission. A woman with varicella at term should not have contact with her child until all of her vesicles have dried.

Most adult women (about 95 percent) are immune to varicella because of infection in childhood. The history of varicella, however, is often incorrect because the patient herself does not remember the infection. The serologic tests ELISA or FAMA can be used to document susceptibility. (See Diagnosis, Mother, Serology, p. 47.)

VZIG can be given to susceptible adults to attempt to prevent or reduce the severity of infection. ELISA or FAMA tests for IgG antibody should be used to identify the 5 percent of women who do not have antibody and are at risk. Almost all women with a history of varicella are immune and about 75 percent of women who have no history of varicella are also immune. VZIG should be administered within 72 hours of exposure. The usual dose for an adult is 5 vials (625 units) and the cost is about $400. Unfortunately, insufficient data are available on the efficacy of VZIG for reducing the severity of varicella in adults and for protecting the fetus from damage.

Vaccines for varicella are under investigation and are being tested in nonpregnant patients who are at high risk for severe disease. There is considerable concern about administration of this vaccine to the general population because the virus might become latent and behave in an unusual way when administered parenterally.

Child

VZIG should be used for the prevention of severe disseminated infection in the child when the mother has chickenpox in the last five days of pregnancy or within 48 hours of delivery. (See Management, Child, p. 49.)

Contact and respiratory isolation procedures should be used for children with chickenpox.

QUESTIONS AND ANSWERS

1. *Should a pregnant woman who is exposed to varicella receive VZIG?*

   The great majority (95%) of pregnant women have had varicella in childhood and are immune. ELISA or FAMA tests are available and should be used to determine if the woman has antibody. VZIG can be given to susceptible women to attempt to suppress the infection. No information is available, however, as to the value of this approach for the protection of the fetus.

2. *If the mother has varicella at term will VZIG given to the child protect it?*

   VZIG should be given to the child when the mother has varicella within the 5 days before delivery or within 48 hours after delivery. The protection is not complete and the child may have some lesions. There is one report of a child who received VZIG and was not protected.

SELECTED READINGS

Centers for Disease Control, U.S. Dept. H.H.S. Varicella-zoster immune globulin distribution—United States and other countries, 1981–1983. *Morbidity and Mortality Weekly Report* 33:81–104, 1984.

Higa, K., et al. Varicella-zoster virus infections during pregnancy: hypothesis concerning the mechanisms of congenital malformations. *Obstet. Gynecol.* 69(2):214–222, 1987.

King, S., et al. Fatal varicella-zoster infection in a newborn treated with varicella-zoster immunoglobulin. *Pediatr. Infect. Dis.* 5(5):588–589, 1986.

Landsberger, E., et al. Successful management of varicella pneumonia complicating pregnancy—a report of three cases. *J. Reprod. Med.* 31(5):311–314, 1986.

Leclair, J., et al. Airborne transmission of chickenpox in a hospital. *N. Engl. J. Med.* 302(8):450–453, 1980.

McGregor, J., et al. Varicella zoster antibody testing in the care of pregnant women exposed to varicella. *Am. J. Obstet. Gynecol.* 157:281–284, 1987.

Paryani, S., and Arvin, A. Intrauterine infection with varicella-zoster virus after maternal varicella. *N. Engl. J. Med.* 314(24):1542–1546, 1986.

Sever, J., and White, L. Intrauterine viral infections. *Ann. Rev. Med.* 19:471–486, 1968.

Stagno, S., et al. Herpesvirus infections of pregnancy. Part II: Herpes simplex virus and varicella-zoster virus infections. *N. Engl. J. Med.* 313(21):1327–1330, 1985.

6

Hepatitis B

The detection of an antigen associated with serum hepatitis (hepatitis B) was first reported in 1968. This methodology has made it possible to identify hepatitis B antigen-positive women and to study the vertical transmission of infection to their babies. Perinatal transmission of hepatitis B from mother to baby is a major life-long health hazard for the infant. Severe late effects (cirrhosis and hepatocellular carcinoma) may be prevented by appropriate immunization of the neonate.

FREQUENCY

Hepatitis B antigen (HB Ag) has been found in approximately 1 of every 1000 adults in the United States and Europe. In Southeast Asia, however, HB Ag is present in 4 to 13 percent of the population, and 40 to 50 percent of chronic carriers may have acquired infection at birth. The hepatitis B virus (HBV) can be transmitted to the infant if acute hepatitis B develops in the mother during pregnancy, particularly when infection is near the time of delivery, or in the first two months post partum. Women with chronic antigenemia can also transmit the infection to children in successive pregnancies.

If the pregnant woman is positive for both hepatitis B surface antigen (HB_sAg) and for hepatitis B e antigen (HB_eAg), the risk of perinatal transmission of hepatitis B to her baby is approximately 80 to 90 percent. Ninety percent of infected infants become chronic carriers of HBsAg. Based on data from Taiwan, approximately 50 percent of the male HB_sAg carriers will die from cirrhosis or primary liver cancer.

If the pregnant woman is only positive for HB_sAg, her expected rate of transmission to the baby falls to 10 to 25 percent. The rate of the HB_sAg carrier state seems to be lower among these infants then if HB_eAg were also present.

Hepatitis D (Delta agent hepatitis) is due to an incomplete RNA virus that depends on coinfection with HBV. When present, the delta agent can cause chronic active hepatitis, cirrhosis, and fulminant hepatitis among patients who are HB_sAg positive. Hepatitis D may also be transmitted perinatally; however, the frequency of this event is not known, in part due to methodologic limitations. The delta agent is usually detectable only in the liver rather than in serum. Nonetheless, a recently developed radioimmunoassay method for detecting antibodies to hepatitis D may permit further epidemiologic study of this form of hepatitis. Testing for IgM antibody to hepatitis D virus may separate those HB_sAg carriers who have underlying inflammatory liver disease due to delta agent from those with resolved or quiescent infection (Farci et al., 1986).

DIAGNOSIS

Mother

Clinical

The incubation period for hepatitis B is variable but is usually 50 to 180 days (Table 6-1). Fever, headache, and abdominal pain may be the initial symptoms. In a few days, as the fever subsides, the urine becomes dark and jaundice appears. The liver is usually enlarged and

Table 6-1. Diagnosis of Hepatitis B

Mother	Child
Clinical	
Blood or secretion exposure Incubation usually 50–180 days Fever, headache, dark urine Jaundice, hepatomegaly	Most asymptomatic, about 10% icteric at 3–4 months of age Rarely death
Laboratory	
Hepatitis B surface antigen (HB_sAg) in blood ALT increased Hepatitis B e antigen (HB_eAg) in blood indicates increased risk for transmission to child	Persisting HB_sAg in blood Some increase in ALT Repeat biopsies show unresolved hepatitis for many months

tender. The spleen is enlarged in about one-fourth of the cases. Jaundice persists for a few days to a month. As the jaundice disappears, the patient feels better and usually recovers rapidly. About 10 percent of patients develop chronic disease. Of this group, 7 percent progress to chronic persistent hepatitis, 3 percent develop chronic active hepatitis, and there are rare cases of fulminant fatal hepatitis.

Laboratory

HB_sAg is present in the blood 30 to 50 days after exposure, and 7 to 21 days before the onset of jaundice. The antigen may disappear with the onset of jaundice or it may persist for many weeks. Chronic HB_sAg carriers occur in about 1 percent of patients in the United States. When antibody to HB_sAg appears, the individual is immune and noninfectious.

The alanine amino transferase (ALT) levels rise about 50 days after exposure and are increased at the time of appearance of jaundice. Abnormal levels of ALT persist for 30 to 60 or more days.

HB_eAg appears early, like HB_sAg. The antigen persists days to weeks, and in some cases indefinitely. When HB_eAg is present, the patient is particularly likely to be infectious by nonparenteral (oral, venereal) as well as parenteral routes. When antibody to e antigen appears (anti-HBe), the patient is much less likely to be infectious.

Child

Clinical

The most frequent response of neonates to hepatitis B infection is asymptomatic chronic hepatitis B (HB_sAg in the blood) with histologic evidence of unresolved hepatitis. Although clinical illness is relatively infrequent with congenital infection, severe disease, including fatal neonatal hepatitis, has been reported. In one study, only 2 of 17 antigen-positive infants showed acute icteric hepatitis, and jaundice appeared at three and four months of age. In rare instances, infants with congenital infection have succumbed from advanced fibrosis of the liver at 1½ years of age.

Table 6-2. Management of Hepatitis B

Mother	Child
Treatment	
Increased rest, symptomatic treatment	Increased rest, symptomatic treatment
High-protein, low-fat diet	No specific treatment
Needle precautions and sterile technique but no isolation	Needle precautions and sterile technique but no isolation
Prevention	
Minimize exposures	Minimize exposures
Definite exposure: HBIG 0.06 ml/kg and repeat in 1 month	Mother with hepatitis B during pregnancy and HB_sAg-positive at term
HB vaccination	HBIG on day of birth (0.5 ml/kg) plus begin HB vaccination

Laboratory

Infected newborns can be diagnosed by demonstrating the presence of HB_sAg in the blood. In addition, most of these infants have mild to moderate elevations of serum transaminase levels. Liver biopsies of the infected children may show unresolved hepatitis.

In rare cases of acute icteric hepatitis, there is rapid disappearance of HB_sAg and the development of hepatitis B antibody (HB_sAb).

MANAGEMENT

Mother

No specific treatment is available for hepatitis (Table 6-2). Increased bed-rest periods are often prescribed, particularly after meals. High-protein, low-fat diets are generally recommended. In most studies, the prognosis for patients was not improved by enforcement of extensive bed rest requirements. Needle precautions and sterile technique with wounds or blood should be used, but isolation is not necessary. Patients with other illnesses may require more rest. Resumption of activity for those who are symptom-free can be based on the following liver function tests: (1) ALT levels normal on three successive days, and (2) serum bilirubin level below 2.0 mg/100ml.

Child

Prevention is the best management for the child. (See Prevention, Child, p. 56.) No treatment is indicated for asymptomatic carrier infants. For symptomatic children, supportive care should be given. The use of steroids and HB_sAb has not been of value for treatment. Needle precautions and sterile technique with wounds or blood should be used, but there is no need for strict isolation.

PREVENTION

Mother

The risk of acquiring hepatitis B is greatest for persons who are exposed to hepatitis patients or blood containing HB_sAg. The most evident risk involves household or hospital exposures but includes inoculation of drug users with contaminated needles.

A "definite exposure" is an accidental inoculation with a contaminated needle or close, physical contact (including sexual contact) that may enhance transmission of blood or secretions. Women who have had a definite exposure to HBV should be given hepatitis B immune globulin (HBIG). In a dose of 0.06 ml/kg as soon as possible (preferably within 24 hours) after exposure. For those women who appear at risk for repeated HB_sAg exposure, it is recommended that a course of HB vaccine be started as soon as possible within seven days of exposure. If HB vaccine has not been given, a second dose of HBIG should be given. HBIG alone is expected to be about 75 percent effective, 25 to 30 days after the first dose.

Specific recommendations to minimize exposures include the following:

Hospitals—General Areas

Patients with acute hepatitis or HB_sAg need not be isolated, providing that attendants take special precautions when handling blood or blood-contaminated objects. These precautions include using gloves and possibly protective clothing. Disposable needles and sterile techniques should be used, and adequate sterilization and chemical disinfection procedures are important. Masks should be worn if there is a chance of splattering blood. Breaks in the skin should be bandaged carefully. Some hospitals call this *needle precautions* and maintain these procedures until HB_sAg is no longer detected and the patient is improving clinically.

Hepatitis—Special Areas

Hemodialysis units are a great risk to patients and staff. Most infections are subclinical and many are chronic. Susceptible pregnant women should be excluded from these areas if at all possible. It is desirable that women working in these areas complete their HB vaccination program prior to becoming pregnant.

Laboratories

Hematology, serology, clinical chemistry, autopsy, and hepatitis research laboratories are well-known risk areas for HBV. Accidental skin puncture by contaminated instruments, mouth pipetting, and contamination of cuts, scratches, eyes, or mouth are likely routes of inoculation. Laboratory rules should restrict mouth pipetting, smoking, eating, open centrifuging, and open homogenizing. Gloves and other protective clothing should be used.

Direct Exposure

Several routes of exposure to HBV have been documented and should be avoided:

1. Direct percutaneous inoculation of contaminated blood or blood products
2. Non-needle transfer of infected blood or blood products through minute skin cuts or abrasions
3. Inadvertent introduction into buccal or ocular surfaces
4. Introduction of infected saliva or semen into mucosal surfaces through sexual contact
5. Transfer through fomites such as shared razors, toothbrushes, towels, washcloths, or similar personal items

An inactivated vaccine (Heptavax-B) has been developed from the surface antigen of hepatitis B virus. Its use is recommended for physicians, nurses, and laboratory personnel who are likely to come into contact with infectious patients, or specimens or secretions from such patients. Since the hepatitis B virus has been isolated from blood, amniotic fluid, urine, vaginal secretions, and breast milk, the staff and students associated with obstetrics and newborn care are considered at risk for exposure. HB vaccination for healthy adults involves a sequence of three intramuscular injections (1.0 ml each) with the second and third injections given at one month and six months following the first. HB vaccination may be started at the time HBIG is given for an acute exposure without a decrease in vaccine effectiveness. Pregnancy does not contraindicate vaccination among otherwise eligible women.

Child

Women who have hepatitis B during pregnancy can transmit the infection to their children. The risk is greatest in the last trimester of pregnancy and first two months post partum. In some cases, the virus infects the child in utero and at birth the child is already HB_sAg positive. In most instances the child is exposed at delivery or in the first weeks of life. The sources of exposure include (1) ingestion of blood and inoculation through abrasions at delivery, (2) ingestion of blood and infected milk while nursing, (3) exposure to mother's secretions by direct contact, (4) inoculation through delivery monitoring procedures, and (5) injections that may penetrate the newborn's skin, which is contaminated with the virus.

Children born to women who have hepatitis B during pregnancy and who are HB_sAg positive at term should be given HBIG within 12 hours of birth in a single dose of 0.5 ml intramuscularly. The efficacy of HBIG is expected to decline sharply if there is a delay in administration beyond 48 hours. A 3-dose series of HB vaccine should be started within seven days of birth (0.5 ml intramuscularly). Repeat doses should be given at one and six months. The combination of HBIG and HB vaccine is expected to be about 90 percent effective in preventing infants from becoming HB_sAg carriers. A program of serologic testing at 6 to 15 months of age will identify the treatment failures (carriers) and allow specific counseling.

If the mother develops hepatitis after delivery, the child should be given HBIG as indicated for a definite exposure. To minimize transmission of infection from the infected mother to the child, women should be instructed on careful handwashing. If the skin on the mother's hands is excoriated, she should use disposable gloves when caring for the child. Children who are infected and in the hospital should be placed on needle precautions and sterile technique should be used with blood. Complete isolation is not necessary but some hospitals isolate infected newborns with the antigen-positive mothers.

Since HBV has been isolated from breast milk, milk from an HB_sAg mother must be regarded as a potential source of transmission of infection. Breast feeding can be permitted if the immunization program recommended above has been used. Avoiding breast feeding does not by itself eliminate the risk of hepatitis B for the infant, since there are so many other ways for the virus to be transmitted.

Since immunization of newborns is highly effective in preventing perinatal transmission of HBV, and since it is desirable to minimize infectious risks for health care workers, a screening program should be used to detect HB_sAg in pregnant women. In the United States, routine screening of all pregnant women has been recommended by the Centers for Disease Control (1988). This testing should be done during an early prenatal visit at the same time that other routine prenatal screening tests are ordered. If the prenatal screen was not done, it should be accomplished at delivery.

In parts of the world where HBV infection is highly endemic, universal vaccination of newborns is recommended to minimize both perinatal and childhood acquisition of HBV. In these areas, vaccination of newborns may represent a better use of available resources than prenatal HB_sAg screening.

OTHER TYPES OF HEPATITIS

Hepatitis A (infectious hepatitis) has not been found to be associated with fetal or newborn disease. Pregnant women and children with household or other short-duration exposure should be given ISG, 0.02 to 0.05 ml/kg, within two weeks following exposure to provide protection for five to six months.

Non-A non-B hepatitis has become the most frequent cause of transfusion-related hepatitis in many hospitals today. Recent studies suggest that this type of hepatitis behaves similarly to hepatitis B and can be transmitted from mother to child when acute illness occurs in the third trimester of pregnancy. Management should be similar to that described above.

QUESTIONS AND ANSWERS

1. *Should gamma globulin be used for a woman who has had a definite exposure to hepatitis B?*

   Yes. HBIG should be given as soon as possible and within 24 hours of percutaneous exposure. This should be repeated in 25 to 30 days if HB vaccine was not given.

2. *Can hepatitis B be transmitted in utero?*

   Yes, approximately 5 percent of cases occur in utero, but transmission also occurs at the time of birth or shortly thereafter.

3. *Should a C-section be used to avoid infection of the child if the mother has hepatitis B and HB_sAg?*

   No. At present there is no information to indicate this will decrease the exposure of the child to the virus. The child should be given HBIG and HB vaccine as described above.

SELECTED READINGS

Ahtone, J., and Maynard, J. Laboratory diagnosis of hepatitis B. *J.A.M.A.* 249:2067–2069, 1983.

Beasley, R. et al. Prevention of perinatally transmitted hepatitis B virus infections with hepatitis B immune globulin and hepatitis B vaccine. *Lancet* 2:1099–1102, 1983.

Centers for Disease Control, U.S. Dept. H.H.S. Postexposure prophylaxis for hepatitis B. *Morbidity and Mortality Weekly Report* 33(21): 285–290, 1984.

Centers for Disease Control, U.S. Dept. H.H.S. Prevention of perinatal transmission of hepatitis B virus: Prenatal screening of all pregnant women for hepatitis B surface antigen. *Morbidity and Mortality Weekly Report* 37(22):341–351, 1988.

Farci, P. et al. Diagnostic and prognostic significance of the IgM antibody to the hepatitis delta virus. *J.A.M.A.* 255:1443–1446, 1986.

Sever, J., and White, L. Intrauterine viral infections. *Ann. Rev. Med.* 19:471–486, 1968.

Snydman, D. Hepatitis in pregnancy. *N. Engl. J. Med.* 313:1398–1401, 1985.

Stevens, C., et al. Yeast-recombinant hepatitis B vaccine: Efficacy with hepatitis B immune globulin in prevention of perinatal hepatitis B virus transmission. *J.A.M.A.* 257:2612–2616, 1987.

Tong, M., et al. Studies on the maternal-infant transmission of viruses which cause acute hepatitis. *Gastroenterology.* 80:999–1004, 1986.

Wong, V. et al. Prevention of the HB_sAg carrier status in newborn infants in mothers who are chronic carriers of HB_sAg and HB_eAg by administration of hepatitis B vaccine and hepatitis B immune globulin: double-blind randomized placebo-controlled study. *Lancet* 1:921–926, 1984.

7

Influenza

Epidemics of febrile respiratory disease clinically recognized as influenza have been known for more than 100 years. During major epidemics, the infection has been associated with significant increases in morbidity and mortality. Maternal mortality can be due to pneumonia or to exacerbation of a preexisting cardiopulmonary condition or other chronic disorder. Although there are three antigenically distinct types of influenza viruses, most epidemics and severe cases are due to type A. Type B influenza virus generally causes milder disease. Type C influenza virus is the least significant.

FREQUENCY

The frequency and severity of influenza epidemics have been related to antigenic changes in the virus. Minor antigenic changes have been reported annually, while major changes have come at 10- to 30-year intervals. In general, major antigenic changes have been associated with more severe illness related to presumed increased numbers of susceptible individuals in the population.

It is well established that chronically ill adults, children, and elderly persons are high-risk individuals for major morbidity related to influenza. On the other hand, pregnancy without concurrent chronic illness is not considered a high-risk factor for morbidity due to influenza. Some reports, particularly from major epidemics (1918–19 and 1957–58), have identified increased mortality among pregnant or puerperal women; however, other reports have not supported that conclusion. Pneumonia is a major complication of influenza, either as primary viral or secondary bacterial infection, which can be fatal. Maternal mortalities related to influenza have occurred predominantly among women who also had pneumonia. The pneumonia due to the influenza virus may be particularly likely in the gravida who also has prior cardiovascular disease. If bacterial pneumonia occurs, the organism most often isolated is the *Streptococcus pneumoniae* but other streptococci as well as *Staphylococcus aureus* and *Escherichia coli* and other gram-negative rods may be expected.

The effect of maternal influenza on the fetus has not been resolved. The virus has been reported to cross the placenta from mother to fetus but apparently is a rare occurrence. Even in cases of overwhelming maternal infection, the virus may be absent from the fetal compartment.

A miscellaneous group of birth defects has been reported in the offspring of women with histories that suggested maternal influenza during the first trimester. No specific pattern of damage has been consistently noted, although some studies primarily have considered neural tube defects. Maternal influenza during pregnancy is very unlikely to be the direct cause of a congenital malformation, and the influenza virus is not considered to be a proven teratogen.

The newborn is susceptible to influenza except as protected by passive transfer of maternal IgG antibodies and relative seclusion from exposure beyond the nursery or family situation. Premature newborns may be more susceptible to influenza than term babies; however, part of the apparent susceptibility may be due to respiratory compromise rather than any more general impairment of immune mechanisms.

Table 7-1. Diagnosis of Influenza

Mother	Child
Clinical	
Fever (can reach 39° C) Malaise (can progress to prostration) Myalgias Conjunctivitis Sore throat and cough Pulmonary findings limited to scattered rales and rhonchi unless pneumonia is present	Indistinguishable from bacterial sepsis (See Chap. 16, Neonatal Sepsis)
Laboratory (Mother and Child)	
Specific	Nonspecific
Virus isolation Serology (seroconversion or 2-tube increased titer) Complement fixation Hemagglutination inhibition	Erythrocyte sedimentation rate increased CBC may show leukopenia Chest x-ray: no change unless pneumonia is present

DIAGNOSIS

Mother

Influenza becomes manifest as upper respiratory infection of varying severity accompanied by fever, malaise, myalgias, and headache following an incubation period of less than one to four days (Table 7-1). Usually the major portion of clinical disease lasts for three days or less; however, the recovery to a general feeling of well-being and full activity may take a variable course over several days. Physical examination of an uncomplicated patient can at most demonstrate erythema of the pharynx and conjunctiva, and scattered rales or rhonchi in addition to pyrexia.

Routine clinical laboratory findings are unremarkable when influenza is uncomplicated. The chest x-ray remains clear. Definitive diagnosis can be made by virus isolation from throat washings obtained during the first three days of illness or by serologic demonstration of a two-tube or greater rise in antibodies. Either complement fixation (CF) or hemagglutination inhibition (HI) tests may be done to test for development of antibodies.

Child

The clinical manifestations of influenza in the newborn are indistinguishable from those due to sepsis in general. (See Chap. 16, Neonatal Sepsis.) Definitive laboratory diagnosis depends on virus isolation and serologic testing as in adults. Owing to the overlap of manifestations with bacterial sepsis, the diagnosis of influenza in the newborn is neither expected nor possible unless such specific diagnostic studies are done. Usually suggestive circumstances, such as a known influenza epidemic in the adult community or nursery itself, would be required before such studies would be ordered.

Table 7-2. Influenza Management

Mother	Child
Uncomplicated Rest Liberal oral fluid intake Acetaminophen tablets 325–650 mg orally 3–4 times daily For relief of severe coughing, codeine 7.5–30 mg may be given orally every 4 hours	See Chap. 16, Neonatal Sepsis
Complicated by pneumonia If smear of sputum or tracheal aspirate shows gram-positive lancet-shaped diplococci, use penicillin G, IV, usually 2–4 million units/day in divided doses. Dosage may be increased to 20–30 million units per day when treating overwhelming infection If smear of sputum or tracheal aspirate is inconclusive or if *S. aureus* is suspected, use nafcillin, IV, 6 g/day in 6 divided doses (some authorities recommend using up to 12 g/day for the most severe cases) If smear of sputum or tracheal aspirate shows gram-negative rods or if gram-negative bacteria are suspected, add to penicillin or nafcillin the following: gentamicin, IV, 3–5 mg/kg/day in 3–4 divided doses	
High-risk patients with influenza Add amantadine 200 mg/day PO. May be given in 2 divided doses	

MANAGEMENT

Mother

Since the usual course of influenza is self-limited and not altered by antibiotics, therapy is directed toward symptomatic relief (Table 7-2). Bedrest at home with liberal oral fluid intake is a reasonable policy. Acetaminophen may be recommended for fever and myalgias. For severe coughing, codeine may also be given.

The obstetrician should be vigilant for possible pneumonia as a complication. Pneumonia is best treated in the hospital. Intravenous antibiotics are needed and should be directed to cover the broad spectrum of possible secondary bacterial infection unless more specific therapy may be selected based on Gram's stain or culture of the sputum or tracheal aspirate. The details of the management of respiratory therapy for deteriorating pulmonary function requires appropriate consultation. Management should include precautions to protect the patient from nosocomial bacterial infection as well as to protect others in the hospital from influenza. In general, the management plan should not include induction of labor or elective cesarean section while pneumonia is present, unless other obstetrical considerations mandate such a course. If delivery requires more extensive anesthesia than local infiltration or block, an anesthesiology consultation should be sought in an effort to provide optimal pain relief with a minimum of added respiratory compromise. Epidural anesthesia is usually preferred.

In nonpregnant patients, the antiviral drug amantadine has been used for both treatment and prophylaxis of influenza A. In patients who were symptomatic before starting the drug, studies have shown improved pulmonary function and reduced duration of fever. However, the drug has not been studied in pregnant women, and very high doses have been teratogenic and embryotoxic for rats. Therefore,

Table 7-3. Influenza Prevention

Mother	Child
Annual immunization with inactivated virus preparation Nonepidemic: only high-risk patients Epidemic: any pregnant woman not allergic to eggs Amantadine prophylaxis for high-risk patients not vaccinated Nonepidemic: 200 mg/day PO for 10 days following known exposure to influenza Epidemic: 200 mg/day PO for up to 3 months. Immunize, unless patient has egg allergy. Amantadine prophylaxis may be stopped 2–3 weeks after immunization	During epidemics minimize exposure by prior immunization of mothers, physicians, nurses, and other staff members Neither direct immunization nor amantadine has been used in newborns

use of amantadine for pregnant women would need to be limited to those extraordinary cases in which influenza appears to be life-threatening. Since the drug appears in breast milk, the same criteria for therapy would apply to breast-feeding women. Amantadine does not have any beneficial effect against influenza B.

Child

Manage as for bacterial septicemia. (See Chap. 16, Neonatal Sepsis.)

PREVENTION

Under normal circumstances annual immunization against influenza is advised for only high-risk individuals such as the chronically ill or elderly (Table 7-3). These criteria exclude the vast majority of pregnant women; however, vaccination is appropriate for those pregnant women who have a significant medical complication of pregnancy that acts to limit cardiovascular, pulmonary, or immune function. Examples would include congenital heart disease, rheumatic heart disease, tuberculosis, severe asthma, bronchiectasis, chronic renal disease with azotemia or nephrotic syndrome, insulin-dependent diabetes, cystic fibrosis, neuromuscular or orthopedic disorders that impair ventilation, and sickle cell anemia. In order to anticipate winter and spring seasonal influenza epidemics, the optimal time for vaccination is November. Earlier vaccination may be appropriate if local circumstances lead to expecting an earlier influenza season or unavailability of the patient for November vaccination. It may be reasonable to delay vaccination of a pregnant woman in the first trimester as a precaution to minimize concern regarding the theoretical possibility of a teratogenic effect, provided the delay does not substantially increase the risk of maternal acute influenza. Since the vaccines in current use are formulations of inactivated viruses, the risk of malformation due to first-trimester exposure is negligible.

Common minor side effects may include local soreness at the inoculation site, fever, malaise, and myalgia. Rare allergic responses to the egg protein in the influenza vaccine occur and may include anaphylaxis. Persons with known allergic hypersensitivity to eggs should *not* be vaccinated. An additional possible, and severe, complication of influenza vaccination is the Guillain-Barré syndrome, a usually self-limited and reversible disorder in which ascending paralysis is the most prominent feature. The approximate incidence of Guillain-Barré syndrome was 10 cases for every million persons vaccinated in the 1976 swine influenza vaccination program. An increased risk of Guillain-Barré syndrome has not been associated with influenza A vaccination programs in subsequent years.

In years of epidemic influenza, vaccination programs usually are expanded to include the general population rather than only high-risk susceptible people. During such an epidemic control program, pregnant women should be vaccinated, too. There is no evidence that pregnant women have any more adverse effects from vaccination with inactivated virus than nonpregnant women.

As amantadine may uncommonly be used in treatment of influenza in certain high-risk pregnant patients, it might also be used for prophylaxis of such patients who have not been vaccinated (Table 7-3). The drug should be started as soon as possible before or immediately after exposure. Prophylaxis should be maintained by daily dosage until the risk of influenza exposure has passed (up to three months) or until vaccination has become effective (two to three weeks).

QUESTIONS AND ANSWERS

1. *If influenza has been diagnosed during the first half of pregnancy, should an amniocentesis be performed to assess fetal condition?*

   No. Influenza is not expected to have a significant adverse effect on the fetus.

2. *Should a pregnant woman who has influenza be given routine antibiotic coverage?*

   No. Indiscriminate antibiotic use can lead to emergence of resistant bacteria and allergic reactions.

SELECTED READINGS

Centers for Disease Control, U.S. Dept. H.H.S. Prevention and control of influenza. *Morbidity and Mortality Weekly Report.* 35(20):317–326, 1986.

Finland, M. Influenza. In D. Charles and M. Finland (Eds.), *Obstetrics and Perinatal Infections*. Philadelphia: Lea and Febiger, 1973. Pp. 355–398.

Mackenzie, J., and Houghton, M. Influenza infections during pregnancy: Association with congenital malformations and subsequent neoplasms in children, and potential hazards of live virus vaccines. *Bacteriol. Rev.* 38:356–370, 1974.

Meibaline, R., et al. Outbreak of influenza in a neonatal intensive care unit. *J. Pediatr.* 91:974–976, 1977.

Ramphal, R., Donelly, W., and Small, P. Fatal influenzal pneumonia in pregnancy: Failure to demonstrate transplacental transmission of influenza virus. *Am. J. Obstet. Gynecol.* 138:347–348, 1980.

Sumaya, C., and Gibbs, R. Immunization of pregnant women with influenza A/New Jersey/76 virus vaccine: Reactogenicity and immunogenicity in mother and infant. *J. Infect. Dis.* 140:141–146, 1979.

Warrell, M., Tobin, J., and Wald, N. Examination for influenza IgA and IgM antibodies in pregnancies associated with fetal neural tube defects. *J. Med. Microbiol.* 14:159–162, 1981.

8

Human Papillomavirus Infections (Condylomata Acuminata)

Condylomata acuminata are genital warts histologically composed of papillomatous growths of epithelial cells (Fig. 8-1). These cells characteristically contain intranuclear inclusion bodies. When studied by electron microscopy, some of these inclusion bodies have been found to contain papovavirus-like particles. Presently, human papillomavirus, a member of subgroup A of the family Papovaviridae, is considered to be the causative agent of human genital warts. Human papillomavirus (HPV) is an icosadeltahedral viral particle, 45 to 55 nanometers in diameter. The viral genome is composed of circular, double-stranded DNA. Genital warts have been described since classical times and considered a form of sexually transmitted disease since antiquity. This view was not proved, however, until 1954, when studies of servicemen returning from the Korean War provided substantiation. HPV was first identified by electron microscopy in human genital tissue in 1968.

FREQUENCY

HPV infections are relatively common among sexually active individuals. Seventy-five percent of all adults have antibodies suggestive of prior infection. Although condylomata are not considered to be a reportable disease, estimates of the frequency of infection in the United States are available through other health reporting agencies. The National Disease and Therapeutic Index (NDTI) has reported that the number of U.S. consultative visits for genital warts increased from 169,000 in 1966 to 949,000 in 1981. In the latter year, three times as many individuals sought professional consultation for genital warts as did for herpes simplex virus infections.

Two to ten percent of all women of childbearing age are estimated to have genital warts. In one large prospective study of the prevalence of condylomata acuminata in pregnancy, 3.2 percent of all women screened by urine cytology and confirmed virologically were found to be infected with warts.

Knowledge concerning the natural history of human wart infections is relatively limited. In addition to transfer of infection through sexual contact, clinical evidence suggests that some infections are acquired perinatally. Although a newborn may acquire the virus by contact with infected maternal genital surfaces during parturition, some evidence suggests that cases occur as a result of transplacental (hematogeneous) transfer of infection prior to birth.

DIAGNOSIS

Mother

Genital warts appear as papillomatous excrescences either alone or in clusters on mucous membrane surfaces. Occasionally during pregnancy they may proliferate extensively, causing soft tissue dystocia, necessitating cesarean section delivery in some cases. Recently, evidence has been advanced implicating infection of genital surfaces

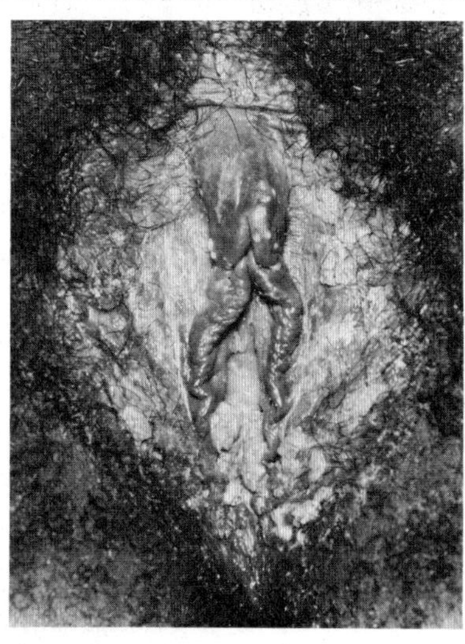

Fig. 8-1. Exophytic lesions of condylomata acuminata.

with certain HPV strains (16 and 18) to subsequent development of cervical carcinoma. Currently, no laboratory tests are available to screen for cells incubating papillomavirus infection.

Subclinical papillomavirus infections may occasionally be detected by exfoliative cytology. Koilocytosis is regarded as the most reliable criterion for diagnosing infection from Papanicolaou smears. Pregnant women whose PAP smears suggest subclinical infection with condylomata acuminata should undergo careful repeat visual and colposcopic examination by individuals with expertise in this area. In selected cases, histologic examination of biopsy samples may be necessary for complete clinical assessment (Table 8-1). The increased vascularity of genital epithelial surfaces during pregnancy makes care and discretion important when determining the timing and extent of such testing during gestation. Immunochemical staining and electron microscopy of histologic specimens may be helpful diagnostic adjuncts in some cases. Papillomavirus DNA probes have recently been developed, and hold promise as future tools for epidemiologic surveillance and as screening and diagnostic approaches.

Child

Newborns may develop genital or perianal condylomata similar to those found in adults. Occasionally, babies develop laryngeal papillomas. These rapidly growing, noninvasive tumors can cause hoarseness, stridor, dyspnea, and acute respiratory obstruction. The frequency with which neonatal laryngeal papillomas occur as a result of prior maternal genital condylomata acuminata is unknown. At least one prospective study of 1,235 pregnant women (of whom 3% were actively infected with warts) suggests that perinatal transmission is low. Nevertheless, numerous case studies suggest an association be-

Table 8-1. Diagnosis of HPV Infections

Mother	Child
Clinical	
Clinical appearance	Clinical appearance Respiratory obstruction (laryngeal papillomas)
Laboratory	
Koilocytosis on Pap smear Histologic studies (if indicated)	Histologic studies (if indicated)

tween neonatal laryngeal papillomas and vaginal birth complicated by genital wart infection. Whether such neonatal infections are preventable by cesarean section delivery is problematic at present. Papillomavirus DNA has been demonstrated in "normal" laryngeal tissue of patients in remission following extirpation of laryngeal lesions. Moreover, laryngeal papillomas develop among individuals of all ages with equal frequency, ranging from 3 months to 70 years of age. These findings suggest that many individuals may acquire subclinical infection of laryngeal tissues at birth. Until more is known about the natural history of HPV infection, no definitive statements can be made about the perinatal implications of maternal genital wart infections or strategies such as cesarean delivery to prevent viral infection of the newborn. There are no prospective studies proving that cesarean section reduces the rate of perinatal transmission of HPV infection. At present, the potentially major surgical complications of cesarean section delivery and the comparative rarity of neonatal laryngeal papillomas makes abdominal delivery for condylomata acuminata a controversial preventative measure on behalf of the child, at best.

MANAGEMENT

Topical application of podophyllum during pregnancy has been associated with significant maternal toxicity and death. Although use of this agent has not been conclusively associated with fetal malformation, isolated reports of perinatal mortality associated with extensive application of this agent have also been reported. For these reasons, podophyllum should *not* be used in pregnancy. Staged local ablation of extensive vulvovaginal condylomata have been successfully performed using electrocautery, cryosurgery, or carbon dioxide laser therapy (Table 8-2). Care must be taken to prevent extensive sloughage or scarring. Like laryngeal papillomas, Southern blot analysis of genital epithelium adjacent to treatment areas has demonstrated the presence of HPV genome in apparently "normal" cells following treatment. Residual subclinical infection may occur in as many as 45 percent of all treated cases. The group of individuals with latent, persistent subclinical disease is six to eight times more likely to develop recurrent infection compared to groups of individuals who, following treatment, are free of evidence of persistent HPV infection at the edges of tissue resection.

Treatment of laryngeal papillomas may be extremely difficult. Re-

Table 8-2. Management of HPV Infections

Mother	Child
Treatment	
Surgical ablation Electrocautery Cryosurgery CO_2 laser ?Interferon	Surgical ablation ?Interferon
Prevention	
Avoid contact with infected individuals	?Cesarean section delivery in some cases

currences are not uncommon and, aside from extirpative surgery, few therapeutic approaches have demonstrated efficacy. Limited trials with immunotherapeutic agents such as interferon are under way and may provide some hope as therapeutic alternatives. Whether the risk of cesarean section delivery is justified in an attempt to prevent neonatal condylomata must await further study.

PREVENTION

Presently, the epidemiology of human HPV infections is not well understood. Until more information concerning the risks of transmission and better methods of detection are available, no meaningful statements concerning prevention of this disease can be made.

SELECTED READINGS

Bergman, A., Bhatia, N., and Broen, E. Cryotherapy for treatment of genital condylomata during pregnancy. *J. Repro. Med.* 29:432–435, 1984.

Centers for Disease Control, U.S. Dept. H.H.S. Condyloma acuminatum—United States, 1966–1981, *Morbidity and Mortality Weekly Report,* 32:306–308, 1983.

Chamberlain, M., Reynolds, A., and Yeoman, W. Toxic effect of podophyllum application in pregnancy. *Br. Med. J.* 3:391–392, 1972.

Coleman, D., et al. A prospective study of human polyomavirus infection in pregnancy. *J. Infect. Dis.* 142:1–8, 1980.

Cook, T., et al. Laryngeal papilloma: Etiologic and therapeutic considerations. *Ann. Otolaryn.* 82:649–655, 1973.

Ferenczy, A. Treating genital condyloma during pregnancy with the carbon dioxide laser. *Am. J. Obstet. Gynecol.* 148:9–12, 1984.

Ferenczy, A., et al. Latent papillomavirus and recurring genital warts. *N. Engl. J. Med.* 313:784–788, 1985.

Smotkin, D., et al. Human papillomavirus deoxyribonucleic acid in adenosquamous carcinoma and adenosquamous carcinoma of the uterine cervix. *Obstet. Gynecol.* 68:241–244, 1986.

Steinberg, B., et al. Laryngeal papillomavirus infection during clinical remission. *N. Engl. J. Med.* 308:1261–1264, 1983.

Syrjanen, K. Current concepts of human papillomavirus infections in the genital tract and their relationship to intraepithelial neoplasia and squamous cell carcinoma. *Obstet. Gynec. Surv.* 39:252–265, 1984.

Tang, C., Shermeta, D., and Wood, C. Congenital condylomata acuminata. *Am. J. Obstet. Gynecol.* 131:912–913, 1978.

Wilson, J. Extensive vulval condylomata acuminata necessitating cesarean section. *Aust. N. Z. J. Obstet. Gynecol.* 13:121–124, 1973.

Young, R., Acosta, A., and Kaufman, R. The treatment of large condylomata acuminata complicating pregnancy. *Obstet. Gynecol.* 41:65–73, 1973.

Mumps

Mumps is a relatively uncommon infection during pregnancy. For nearly 20 years, a live-attenuated mumps strain has been available for vaccination that has been effective in preventing primary infections. Salter, in 1849, is said to have been the first to report a case of mumps complicating pregnancy. This pregnancy subsequently ended by spontaneous abortion of the fetus.

FREQUENCY

Prior to the advent of vaccination to prevent mumps, this disease characteristically occurred prior to puberty. Mumps virus belongs to the Paramyxoviridae family of viruses that also includes respiratory syncytial virus, parainfluenza viruses, and measles virus. All members of this family of viruses cause infections of the upper respiratory tract in humans. Man is one of the few natural hosts for mumps virus. Less than 10 percent of all naturally occurring mumps occurs after the age of 15, and many adults are immune by virtue of a forgotten or subclinical infection during childhood. As children who were vaccinated following the availability of immunization reach adulthood, it is likely that the pool of susceptible adults will become even smaller. Even among susceptible parents exposed to infected children within the same household, the attack rate is low. Few mothers who lack neutralizing antibodies will contract the disease; therefore, mumps during pregnancy is an uncommon event. Surveys of the incidence of mumps complicating pregnancy have provided a range of estimates of frequency from 0.8 to 10 cases/10,000 deliveries.

DIAGNOSIS

Mother

Mumps virus is generally transmitted in saliva and enters the host following inhalation of droplet contamination. The virus can be recovered from saliva two or three days before and five to seven days after the onset of illness. Clinical disease typically occurs as acute parotitis with fever and malaise approximately 16 to 18 days after exposure (Table 9-1). A viremia precedes clinical symptoms by several days and may persist for up to five days after the onset of salivary gland inflammation. Although a generally self-limited and relatively complication-free disease, mumps can be a significant cause of morbidity. Unilateral sensorineural deafness, meningitis, pancreatitis, oophoritis, and even death have been reported in adult women. There is no evidence that these events are more common in pregnancy. Retrospective studies, however, have suggested that mumps during the first trimester of pregnancy results in an approximately 2-fold increase in the incidence of spontaneous abortion. A recent report of mumps complicating first trimester pregnancy has demonstrated the transplacental distribution of virus coincident with maternal viremia. Histologic examination of the products of conception following maternal infection in the first trimester demonstrated proliferative necrotic vilitis and necrosis of fetal viscera with inclusions in infected cells suggestive of intrauterine infection.

Usually the clinical picture of mumps is sufficiently characteristic

Table 9-1. Diagnosis of Mumps

Mother	Child
Clinical	
Parotitis	Parotitis
Fever	Fever
Malaise	Malaise
	?Endocardial fibroelastosis
Laboratory	
Viral isolation	Viral isolation
Hemagglutination inhibition	Hemagglutination inhibition
Complement fixation	Complement fixation

to permit the diagnosis on the basis of presenting signs and symptoms alone. Occasionally a subclinical or atypical case will arise, and in such an instance the diagnosis may be confirmed by isolation of the virus or immunulogic testing. Virus isolation may be accomplished by culturing of the oropharynx and utilization of a rhesus monkey kidney cell line. Confirmation of mumps virus infection is accomplished by neutralization with mumps-specific antisera in tissue culture and demonstration that parainfluenza antisera does not inhibit virus growth. Alternatively, serologic testing may be employed. An increase in the soluble (S-nucleocapsid) titer is common early in disease and is followed later by a rise in V antibody (surface hemagglutinin) titer. Complement fixation tests become positive after 14 days. Due to the high incidence of antigenic cross-reactivity, such testing should be conducted with appropriate controls for other related paramyxoviruses. Skin testing, which assesses delayed hypersensitivity, is evidence of immunity but is not reliable when seeking to document an acute infection.

Child

There have been several recent reports concerning the perinatal outcome of acute mumps infections complicating pregnancies at term. In general, the maternal course of the disease has been relatively benign. Several infants have been reported to have been born within one week of the onset of acute maternal infection. Presumably, these infants became infected as a result of hematogenous dissemination of virus during maternal viremia. A wide range of neonatal outcomes, extending from relatively asymptomatic neonatal infection to serious pneumonitis, has occurred. The extent of maternal disease does not appear to predict the severity of neonatal infection.

The predominant concern during the past 15 years has been a possible association between maternal mumps and the development of subsequent congenital cardiac abnormality in neonates, specifically endocardial fibroelastosis (EFE). In the early 1960s, several reports were published suggesting that a high proportion of children clinically diagnosed as having EFE had positive mumps skin tests although they lacked circulating humoral antibody, suggesting that intrauterine infection had occurred. An association between congenital mumps and EFE was proposed. The theory gained some credence when subsequent reports demonstrated that offspring of women exposed to mumps during pregnancy could develop delayed hypersensitivity as demonstrated by a positive mumps skin test in the absence of circulating humoral antibody, implying that intrauterine infection might have occurred. This immunologic phenomenon can be reproduced in the rhesus monkey during pregnancy as well; however, cardiac lesions suggestive of EFE have never been described in this species. Cardiac lesions similar to EFE have been induced in chick embryos exposed to mumps early in development.

Subsequent studies have failed to verify an association between a positive mumps skin test and EFE. Moreover, children with a diagnosis of EFE and a positive mumps skin test who are exposed to mumps contract the disease, suggesting that the skin test may be a false positive. It is possible that the skin test may be a manifestation of previous exposure to another antigenically similar member of the paramyxovirus family; however, serologic assessment of such infants has not suggested the presence of other paramyxovirus infections. Attempts to isolate mumps virus from children with EFE have been unsuccessful. As of now, only one child with EFE has been prospectively identified by observing mothers with documented mumps in pregnancy. If the association is valid, the low incidence of mumps during pregnancy and the infrequent association between EFE and congenital mumps would make this occurrence an extremely infrequent event.

Other isolated instances of congenital corneal opacities and chorioretinitis in human pregnancy have been reported in association with maternal mumps. Aqueductal stenosis with hydrocephalus has been reported in young children following mumps, and a similar congenital lesion can be induced in litters of pregnant hamsters infected with the virus. Nevertheless, similar congenital central nervous system lesions have never been reported in children whose mothers had mumps during pregnancy. In two large reviews of mumps in pregnancy, comprising 1,000 cases, no increases in congenital abnormalities or fetal complications were noted. No conclusive proof has ever been given linking prenatal mumps to any specific congenital defect. Nevertheless, recent experience unequivocally documents the transplacental passage of mumps virus in human pregnancy. Although this experience has been limited to only several cases, histopathologic evidence now suggests that mumps virus can infect and damage developing human embryonic tissue. The likelihood of this event, however, appears to be low.

PROGNOSIS IF UNTREATED

There is currently no treatment of demonstrated efficacy for mumps either in pregnant or nonpregnant patients. Nevertheless, the usual consequences for both mother and child are benign. Exceptions include occasional severe infections in the mother and one case report documenting severe pneumonitis in a newborn following perinatal maternal infection.

MANAGEMENT

Mumps during pregnancy may be managed symptomatically in the majority of cases (Table 9-2). The disease is less contagious than measles or chickenpox. Since mumps is spread by aerosolized droplet

Table 9-2. Management of Mumps in Pregnancy

Mother	Child
Treatment	
Symptomatic	Symptomatic
Respiratory isolation for one week following onset of symptoms	Respiratory isolation for one week following onset of symptoms
Rarely, if ever, an indication for interruption of pregnancy	?Passive immunotherapy in selected cases
Mumps vaccination during pregnancy is contraindicated	
Prognosis	
Usually good	Usually good

contamination, respiratory isolation is appropriate in hospitalized patients during the first week following development of symptoms. On the basis of the information available at present, maternal mumps infection is not itself an indication for interruption of pregnancy. On the other hand, each patient with mumps in pregnancy should be given the information now available about the disease and allowed to consider the alternatives for herself.

In the case report involving an infant suffering perinatal mumps pneumonitis, passive immunotherapy with immune serum globulin was administered. The benefits of this approach are difficult to assess based on a single case. Serologic studies that were performed demonstrated that passive immunization did not interfere with development of an immune response by this baby. Although the value of immune serum globulin for passive immunization of newborns with moderately severe perinatal mumps infections has not been established, it might be considered under some circumstances in selected cases.

PREVENTION

Since the advent of vaccination for mumps nearly 20 years ago, the frequency of naturally occurring mumps infection has steadily declined. Mumps vaccination induces protective antibodies in 95 percent of all susceptible people who are vaccinated without clinically adverse reactions. Although the duration of antibody persistence and protection afforded by immunization is unknown, it appears to parallel naturally induced immunity.

Attenuated virus particles have been recovered from placental tissue of susceptible women vaccinated during pregnancy. As with all live vaccines, immunization is therefore contraindicated during pregnancy on theoretical grounds of potential harm to the developing fetus. Although no damage has ever been demonstrated, the apparently innocuous nature of the disease itself during pregnancy makes assumption of any risk from vaccination, no matter how slight, unwarranted.

SELECTED READINGS

Garcia, A., et al. Intrauterine infection with mumps virus. *Obstet. Gynecol.* 56:756–759, 1980.

Jones, J., Ray, C., and Fulginiti, V. Perinatal mumps infection. *J. Pediatr.* 96:912–914, 1980.

Kurtz, J., Tomlinson, A., and Pearson, J. Mumps virus isolated from a fetus. *Br. Med. J. (Clin. Res.)* 284:471, 1982.

St. Geme, J., Noren, G., and Adams, P. Proposed embryopathic relation between mumps virus and primary endocardial fibroelastosis. *N. Engl. J. Med.* 275:339–347, 1966.

10

Other Viral Infections

PARVOVIRUSES

The human parvovirus B19 was first recognized in 1975. It has been shown to be the cause of erythema infectiosum (fifth disease), transient arthritis/arthralgia, and most cases of aplastic crises in patients with chronic hemolytic anemias. In pregnant women it has now been associated with increased rates of abortions and stillbirths.

Most parvovirus B19 infections occur among children who are 5 to 15 years old. The prevalence of IgG antibodies to B19 is about 2 to 9 percent in children less than 5 years of age, 15 to 35 percent in children 5 to 18 years old, and 30 to 60 percent in adults. Adults are most frequently infected by exposure to children with the disease. About 80 percent of infected adults develop arthralgias or arthritis. The majority of adult cases have been reported in women.

Erythema infectiosum has an incubation period of 4 to 20 days. About half of the patients first develop malaise, sore throat, coryza, and low-grade fever. The rash begins on the face and spreads to the neck, trunk, buttocks, and extremities of most patients. Facial rash is noted in 50 to 100 percent of the cases as a bright erythematous, macular rash on the malar surface. This results in the "slapped cheek" appearance. On the extremities, the rash is particularly evident on the extensor surfaces. The rash can become papular, vesicular, and occasionally purpuric and usually persists for fewer than 10 days.

An aplastic crisis superimposed on underlying hemolytic anemia usually occurs only once in any patient. Such crises have now been associated with B19 infection. Recent data indicates that 90 percent or more cases of aplastic anemia are due to infection with B19 in patients with sickle cell disease, hereditary spherocytosis, hemoglobin SC disease, thalassemia, pyruvate kinase deficiency, and acquired hemolytic anemias.

Parvovirus infections of various types occur naturally in several species of animals and can cause fetal death or congenital malformations.

Infection during pregnancy with parvovirus B19 has been shown by several groups to be associated with an increased rate of abortion and stillbirth. The infections were documented by the presence of B19 IgM antibodies in the maternal serum, evidence for B19 DNA in fetal tissues, or both. A summary analysis of 16 pregnant women infected by B19 during the first half of pregnancy showed that six had spontaneous abortions. Among five pregnant women infected during the second half of pregnancy, two had stillbirths. Among five pregnant women infected at unknown times during pregnancy, two had spontaneous abortions. Studies of six of the aborted or stillborn fetuses showed that five had hydrops fetalis and one was macerated and had severe ascites. The spontaneous abortions or stillbirths occurred from 1 to 10 weeks after maternal infection.

It appears that B19 infection during pregnancy may or may not infect the fetus. When infection of the fetus does occur it may in some cases cause no damage, while in other instances it can cause hydrops fetalis and death. There have been no reports of congenital anomalies associated with this infection. B19 IgM antibody is detectable in 80 to 90 percent of patients with recent infections.

The management of women with known exposure to B19 infection should ideally include the use of serology to document maternal infection by seroconversion or the development of IgM antibody to B19. Unfortunately, these tests are only available in a few locations, such as the Centers For Disease Control. Also, the IgM test does not always become positive in association with the infection. If the patient develops rash, arthritis, or arthralgia, the diagnosis can be made on the basis of the clinical findings. Present information suggests that perhaps 20 to 40 percent of infected women will have abortions or stillbirths in association with the infection. The fetus can be monitored by maternal serum α-fetoprotein and ultrasound. Fetal anemia can be directly assessed in utero by cordocentesis. It has been suggested that in utero transfusion of the fetus may be useful when severe anemia has been documented.

Prevention of spread of infection from patients with erythema infectiosum is difficult since virus excretion in the secretions is at the highest levels prior to the onset of rash. Patients with aplastic crises, however, are likely to be infectious at the time of their symptoms; therefore, it would be desirable for pregnant women to avoid contact with these patients.

No vaccines or chemotherapy are available for this infection.

WESTERN EQUINE ENCEPHALITIS

Most infections in humans with Western equine encephalitis (WEE) are subclinical, but clinically recognized cases are reported from the western and southwestern parts of the United States. The virus is transmitted by mosquitoes and the reservoir is wild birds. The disease affects both horses and man and should be suspected in individuals with influenza-like disease or meningitis-encephalitis.

Several reports have been published concerning the probable transplacental transmission of WEE. In each case, the mother experienced a febrile illness with headache, malaise, and lethargy three to ten days before delivery. Serologic tests taken two to three weeks later showed elevated titers to WEE. The children were well at birth but at 5 to 6 days of age they had evidence of meningitis including fever, twitching movements, jaundice, lethargy, neck rigidity, and bulging fontanelles. Cerebrospinal fluid examination showed 475 to 700 white cells, elevated protein level, and normal glucose. The central nervous system findings were quite severe initially but improved rapidly, and the children were discharged from the hospital after approximately two weeks. One child had evidence of permanent neurologic damage. Serologic tests showed the development of antibody to WEE in these children. Several other women have been documented to have had WEE one to three days before delivery, and their children have been normal.

Based on these reports it appears that, in rare cases, WEE can be transmitted to the fetus when infection occurs late in pregnancy. Treatment is symptomatic and may include the use of steroids. No vaccines are generally available for humans but experimental vaccines have been prepared. Prevention is best accomplished by elimination of breeding places for mosquitoes.

VENEZUELAN EQUINE ENCEPHALITIS

Infections with Venezuelan equine encephalitis (VEE) in humans have been well documented. Horses and small mammals are the hosts and the virus is transmitted by mosquitoes. Epidemics are related to periods of heavy rain causing a proliferation of insect vectors. Clinically, patients have influenza-like illness and some have signs of encephalitis. Antibodies to VEE develop shortly after onset of illness.

Maternal infection with VEE can result in abortion or congenital malformations in the child. The virus primarily affects developing brain tissue. Infection during the third month of gestation has been associated with stillbirth, microcephalus, microphthalmia, luxation of the hips, and severe hypoplasia of the brain. In two cases, when infection occurred at five months' gestation, the cranial cavities were filled with fluid, almost no cortex remained, and the cerebellum was absent. Similarly, in three cases of maternal infection at the eighth month of gestation, the children at birth had massive destruction of cerebral and cerebellar tissue.

Experimental studies with rhesus monkeys have duplicated the findings in man. Monkey fetuses infected intracerebrally two-thirds of the way through pregnancy developed microencephaly, hydrocephalus, and cataracts.

Treatment for VEE infection is symptomatic. Prevention involves elimination of infected hosts and breeding places for mosquitoes. An experimental vaccine is being used in selected populations.

MEASLES

Measles remains a common, worldwide disease that occurs primarily in children. Since the introduction of vaccines in the United States in 1963, the incidence of measles has been greatly reduced. In most years only 10,000 to 50,000 cases are reported. Measles still occurs in unimmunized individuals, and "mini" outbreaks have been reported among susceptible people even when 95 percent of individuals have been immunized. In the Collaborative Perinatal Research Study, measles was reported in 11 of 30,000 pregnancies (see Sever reference in Selected Readings). Infection during pregnancy may constitute risk to the mother and child.

Mother

Studies of large epidemics of measles have shown increased mortality among pregnant women. The deaths were usually related to pneumonia, and the rates were higher in pregnant than in nonpregnant women. Studies in the United States and Australia have indicated that only rarely is measles during pregnancy associated with pneumonia or other medical problems.

To minimize the risk of measles, pregnant women who are exposed and have no history of measles or immunization for measles should be given immune serum globulin (ISG). The ISG in a dose of 0.25 ml/kg should be administered as soon as possible after exposure, preferably within 72 hours. If this is not possible, ISG given up to seven days after exposure may prevent or at least modify the infection. For completeness, a serum specimen may also be taken at the time of the exposure to determine if the woman has antibody and is immune. The enzyme-linked immunosorbent assay (ELISA) or neutralization tests should be used. In most cases, the report on the serum specimen will not be available until after the ISG is given.

Child

Several investigations have suggested an increased rate of prematurity among the children of women who have measles during pregnancy, particularly when the disease occurs late in gestation. No clear evidence exists, however, of increased rates of abortion or congenital malformations with maternal measles.

Measles, as early as seven days before delivery or up to seven days after delivery, may result in transplacental infection and may produce measles in the child either at delivery or within the first 10 days of life. Transplacental infection occurs in, at most, 30 percent of these infants. The remaining children are not infected and are susceptible to infection later in life. With congenital infections, neonatal death rates have been reported to be as high as 27 percent, apparently from pneumonia. Severe otitis media has also been reported. Premature infants are at greater risk for severe damage or death than are term children. These cases were reported during the preantibiotic era, and no recent reports are available. Measles in the child older than 10 days of age is considered to be acquired and is usually mild.

To prevent congenital measles, ISG should be given to susceptible women as soon as possible after exposure. (See Mother, p. 76.) In addition, children born to women who have measles in the last week of pregnancy or the first week post partum should be given ISG as soon as possible (0.25 ml/kg).

In the United States, measles vaccine is recommended for children at 15 months of age. Newborns and infants who have not yet received the vaccine and are exposed to measles should be given a modifying dose of ISG (0.05 ml/kg).

ECHOVIRUSES

Echoviruses are classified as enteroviruses along with the polio and coxsackieviruses. They are responsible for a variety of illnesses in children and adults, including respiratory disease, rashes, gastroenteritis, conjunctivitis, aseptic meningitis, and pericarditis. There have been a number of reports of acquired neonatal infections caused by many of the 26 echoviruses. Clinical findings associated with these neonatal infections include fever with spenomegaly and lymphadenopathy, macular rashes, diarrhea and vomiting, pneumonitis, otitis media, jaundice, coryza with cough, and aseptic meningitis.

Echovirus infections during pregnancy have not been associated with abortions, stillbirths, premature delivery, or congenital malformations. Two reports, however, appear to demonstrate that congenital echovirus infections can produce severe disease and damage to the child. First, echovirus 14 has been reported to be the cause of a febrile illness that developed in a child at 3 days of age. The child had cyanotic episodes followed by apneic spells. The next day, the child had hypothermia, hepatomegaly, bradycardia, and ecchymosis. The child died on the seventh day of life. Laboratory tests revealed thrombocytopenia and leukopenia as well as severe hepatic necrosis. Echovirus 19 has been reported to be the cause of hepatic necrosis and massive hemorrhage in three neonates. One infant was symptomatic at birth and petechiae were observed as well as ecchymosis and apneic spells. This infant died at approximately three hours of life. Thrombocytopenia was detected and echovirus 19 was isolated from major organs and lymph nodes. Two additional twin infants were normal in the first 3 days of life but became cyanotic and lethargic. Apneic spells subsequently occurred along with jaundice and petechiae. The children died on the eighth and ninth days of life with severe gastroenteric bleeding. They had thrombocytopenia, and echovirus 19 was recovered from the major organs of both children. It appears from these reports that echoviruses 14 and 19 can infect the fetus in the perinatal period and produce severe, fatal multiorgan disease with thrombocytopenia.

No vaccines are available for echovirus infections and no treatment is available.

COXSACKIEVIRUSES

The coxsackieviruses are RNA viruses classified as enteroviruses. There are 23 types of group A coxsackievirus and six types of group B. Except in rare cases, group A coxsackieviruses are not believed to cause significant perinatal illness. Group B coxsackieviruses can cause pleurodynia, meningoencephalitis, and myocarditis.

Pleurodynia (also known as devil's grip or Bornholm disease) may occur in epidemics or sporadic cases, most often during summer and fall seasons in temperate climates. The disease is characterized by the sudden onset of sharp, pleuritic chest pain with varying amounts of pyrexia, cough, malaise, headache, and abdominal pain. A pleural friction rub may be present, but the chest x-ray is usually normal. Occasionally Coxsackie B infection is complicated by meningoencephalitis and rarely by paralysis. Generally the disease is self-limited, and complete recovery is expected without therapy other than nonspecific pain medication.

Transplacental transmission of group B coxsackievirus has been demonstrated, but there are too few reports to clearly define the magnitude of risk to the baby. Based on case reports and serologic studies, coxsackievirus infection of the fetus may cause malformation or impaired function of the heart, brain, pancreas, and urogenital system. Apparently, there are no demonstrable adverse effects on the fetus following the majority of maternal infections, and there is not an association between the severity of maternal disease and fetal outcome.

Although group B coxsackieviruses can cause myocarditis in adults and children, myocarditis seems to be a particularly prominent manifestation of infection in the neonate. The clinical syndrome is hard to distinguish from neonatal pneumonia or sepsis except for the electrocardiographic and clinical evidence of severe myocardial damage. Clinical suspicion leading to diagnosis may be aroused by epidemic pleurodynia in the adult community or by evidence of severe myocardial damage. There is no infection-specific treatment for the myocarditis. Digitalization and other supportive therapy is given for cardiac failure. Although this syndrome is often fatal, those who do survive apparently are capable of full recovery.

Diagnosis of coxsackievirus infection is based on virus isolation from throat or rectal swab and serologic evidence of increasing specific antibody titer during convalescence. Either hemagglutination-inhibition or complement fixation tests may be performed; however, neither is immediately useful during the acute illness since a two- to four-week period is required to demonstrate seroconversion or a significant rise in antibody titer.

Since the usual route for transmission of coxsackievirus infection is believed to involve fecal contamination, hand washing and contact isolation are believed to be the best defenses for epidemic infection. In a nursery, the cohort nursing system would also help decrease the likelihood of infant contact from transmission.

DENGUE

Dengue is an acute febrile illness associated with a morbilliform rash and myalgias from which it derives its lay name, *breakbone fever*.

Illness has been endemic in the Americas for more than 200 years. The disease is caused by a member of the arbovirus family (a flavivirus). There are four serovarieties of dengue virus, all of which have been imported into the United States by travelers who have acquired infection in Mexico, Central America, South America, the Caribbean basin, or Asia. No cases of indigenous transmission of disease have occurred within the continental United States. Outbreaks in endemic areas usually follow rainy periods during which the mosquito vector, *Aedes aegypti,* flourishes.

Dengue may be found wherever its mosquito vector exists. Virtually all islands of the Caribbean have experienced outbreaks of infection, including Puerto Rico and the U.S. Virgin Islands. From 1982 through 1984, outbreaks were reported in El Salvador, Honduras, Colombia, Jamaica, Haiti, Trinidad, Barbados, and Mexico. The latter country reports the most cases from among all countries reporting illness in the Americas each year. The total number of cases reported annually in the Western Hemisphere ranges from 25,000 to 50,000.

Occasionally epidemics develop during seasons when local mosquito activity is high. In 1981, 10,000 people were hospitalized in Cuba and 159 deaths were reported during an outbreak of type 2 infection. In summer 1984, an outbreak at Clark Air Base on Luzon Island in the Republic of the Philippines resulted in 42 confirmed cases of dengue fever necessitating hospitalization of 29 individuals. As was true in this instance, outbreaks can usually be controlled by aerial spraying of malathion to control insect vectors.

From 1977 through 1984, approximately 900 suspected cases of dengue have been imported into the continental United States. Although *Aedes aegypti* is present in the southeastern United States (including Texas, Florida, and the Carolinas), at present, all infections in the United States have been imported from other areas and no secondary cases within this country have developed. Physicians should consider dengue in the differential diagnosis of acutely ill, febrile individuals who are returning from tropical areas. The diagnosis may be established by serology or virologic isolation methods.

Acute infection with dengue virus is characterized by the abrupt onset of fever, headache, myalgias, arthralgias, and, occasionally, hemorrhagic manifestations. Other clinical findings include malaise, chills, gastrointestinal upset, a maculopapular eruption, and personality changes with disorientation. Approximately 10 percent of all cases are complicated by minor hemorrhage or thrombocytopenia. Laboratory findings include leukopenia, thrombocytopenia, lymphocytosis, a prolonged partial thromboplastin time, and elevated fibrin degradation products. Fortunately, severe forms of the disease such as hemorrhagic fever (DHF) and shock syndrome are rare.

Information concerning the consequences of dengue in pregnancy is limited. Studies in Haiti and the Dominican Republic show that half of all children have developed dengue antibody by 2 years of age. During a nonepidemic period of surveillance in the Dominican Republic, paired maternal and cord sera were studied in 54 pregnancies associated with type 2 and 3 illness. The attack rate among pregnant women in this population was estimated to be 6 percent. Antibody levels to dengue were considerably higher in cord blood, suggesting transplacental passive immunization. It has been hypothesized that early antibody acquisition may prevent the hemorrhagic fever and shock syndromes associated with second infections. These rarely occur in infants under 6 months old.

Whether malformations result from first trimester dengue fever is unknown. Congenital anomalies could arise as an indirect consequence of dengue if elevated core body temperature occurred during critical periods of organogenesis. To date, no such cases have been reported. Prevention of dengue rests essentially with controlling the mosquito vector and avoiding endemic areas.

RABIES

Human rabies, most commonly acquired by direct contact with infected saliva during an animal bite, results in a progressive and usually fatal encephalitis if untreated. Due to large-scale domestic animal vaccination programs, the majority of bites by rabid animals comes from wildlife reservoirs. Raccoons, skunks, foxes, and bats are the most common hosts.

Transplacental passage of rabies virus and rabies virus antibody has been demonstrated in a variety of nonhuman mammals. Experience with rabies in human pregnancy is limited; however, the offspring of successfully treated mothers have generally done well. Transplacental distribution of antirabies vaccine has been observed in studies of cord blood of newborns whose mothers were successfully treated for rabies during pregnancy. Although the absolute risk of rabies and rabies therapy to the fetus is unknown, the grave prognosis for an untreated infection in the mother dictates that full therapy be administered whenever she is at risk for contracting the disease.

Whenever possible, the suspected rabid animal should be captured, isolated, and observed for 10 days. Any abnormal behavior or suspected neurologic disease should prompt attempts to confirm rabies in the animal by fluorescent antibody staining of brain tissue. The patient should receive a tetanus booster if needed, and the animal bite should be thoroughly cleansed, preferably with soap and water followed by copious rinsing with a quaternary ammonium salt solution such as benzalkonium chloride.

Both active and passive immunization should be given for bites from suspected rabid animals. Immediate protection is accomplished by administering human rabies immune globulin (HRIG), 20 IU/kg. This agent, available from state health departments or the Centers for Disease Control, is the treatment of choice for pregnant women because it essentially eliminates the 20 to 40 percent incidence of serum sickness associated with the administration of equine antirabies serum. Active immunization should simultaneously be accomplished by administration of human diploid cell vaccine (HDCV). This vaccine, produced by L'Institut Merieux, has been licensed for use in the United States since 1980. Prior to the availability of this vaccine, duck embryo vaccine (DEV) was utilized for active vaccination. DEV required administration of substantially more doses of inactivated vaccine, was associated with more frequent allergic reactions to avian antigens, and was less immunogenic than HDCV. Five 1-ml doses of HDCV are given intramuscularly, with the first dose of HDCV at the time HRIG is administered. Subsequent doses are given at 3, 7, 14, and 28 days after the first dose. Although mild local reactions such as erythema, pain, and itching have been reported in approximately one-fourth of HDCV recipients, other allergic reactions have been rare. Headache, myalgia, and gastrointestinal upset occur in 20 percent of recipients. HDCV administration has not been associated with anaphylaxis. Individuals previously vaccinated with DEV appear to develop adequate antibody titers following revaccination with HDCV.

SMALLPOX

In 1979, an independent scientific commission certified global eradication of smallpox. Six months later, the World Health Organization (WHO) accepted this conclusion, and there is no evidence that smallpox will recur as an endemic disease either as the result of reactivation of latent human infections or from animal reservoirs. At least six laboratories have retained variola virus. These laboratories are located in the Netherlands, South Africa, the United Kingdom, China, the USSR, and the United States. Several laboratory outbreaks of infection have resulted in death of inadvertently infected individuals.

Concern has been raised regarding the possibility of using variola virus for biologic warfare. Many authorities have discounted this possibility, reasoning that the comparatively long incubation period, slow spread, and clinical manifestations of this infection would make selective isolation and vaccination strategies likely to limit the damage inflicted by release of variola even among highly susceptible patient populations. Nevertheless, WHO has stockpiled variola vaccine in the event of a smallpox outbreak. By 1980, all but four countries had stopped requiring international certification of smallpox vaccination. The Global Commission on Smallpox stated that the risk of bacterial warfare did not justify vaccination of the general public. Nevertheless, certain segments of the population continue to be vaccinated against smallpox infection, including laboratory workers who may come in contact with infectious virus and some military personnel. Thus, although smallpox has been eradicated as a naturally occurring disease, vaccination against smallpox continues to be occasionally administered.

Although vaccination is a relatively safe procedure, it is not entirely without risk. Generalized vaccinia, postvaccinial encephalitis, eczema vaccinatum, and even death can complicate primary or repeat vaccination. In one survey from Australia, the rate of adverse reactions to smallpox vaccination was estimated to be 1 in 5000. The death rate, chiefly from postvaccinial encephalitis, was estimated to be 1.5 per million. Generalized vaccinia is the most common adverse reaction. Women appear to be more prone to adverse reactions following vaccination than men. Administration of vaccinia immune globulin (VIG) results in rapid resolution of most adverse vaccine reactions.

Smallpox vaccination should not be given to pregnant women. Intrauterine vaccinia with fetal death can occur in any trimester. Although this most frequently occurs following primary vaccination, it has been described following revaccination as well. Since the mortality due to smallpox complicating pregnancy has been high, in the unlikely event of an epidemic of smallpox, all people including pregnant women should be vaccinated. In this case, the risk of disease would significantly outweigh the risk of fetal damage by vaccination.

SELECTED READINGS

Parvoviruses

Carrington, D., et al. Maternal serum α-fetoprotein—A marker of fetal aplastic crisis during intrauterine human parvovirus infection. *Lancet* 1:433–435, 1987.

Woernle, C., et al. Human parvovirus B19 infection during pregnancy. *J. Infect. Dis.* 156:17–20, 1987.

Western Equine Encephalitis

Copps, S. C., and Giddings, L. E. Transplacental transmission of Western equine encephalitis. *Pediatr.* 24:31–33, 1959.

Shinefield, H. R., and Townsend, T. E. Transplacental transmission of Western equine encephalomyelitis. *J. Pediatr.* 43:21–25, 1953.

Venezuelan Equine Encephalitis

Wenger, F. Venezuelan equine encephalitis. *Teratology* 16(3):359–362, 1977.

Measles

Dyer, I. Measles complicating pregnancy. *Southern Medical Journal* 33(6):601–604, 1940.

Sever, J. L., and White, L. H. Intrauterine viral infections. *Ann. Rev. Med.* 19, 471, 1968.

Echoviruses

Krous, H. F., Dietzman, D., and Ray, C. G. Fatal infections with ECHOvirus types 6 and 11 in early infancy. *Am. J. Dis. Child.* 126:842–846, 1973.

Modlin, J. F. Perinatal ECHOvirus infection: Risk of transmission during a community outbreak. *N. Engl. J. Med.* 305(7):368–371, 1981.

Coxsackieviruses

Baker, D., and Phillips, C. Maternal and neonatal infection with coxsackievirus. *Obstet. Gynecol.* 55 (Suppl. 3): 12S–15S, 1980.

Brown, G., and Karunas, R. Relationship of congenital anomalies and maternal infection with selected enteroviruses. *Am. J. Epidemiol.* 95:207–217, 1972.

Burch, G., et al. Interstitial and coxasackievirus B myocarditis in infants and children, *J.A.M.A.* 203:1–8, 1968.

Kaplan, M., et al. Group B coxsackievirus infections in infants younger than three months of age: A serious childhood illness. *Rev. Infect. Dis.* 5:1019–1032, 1983.

Reyes, M., et al. Coxsackievirus-positive cervices in women with febrile illnesses during the third trimester in pregnancy. *Am. J. Obstet. Gynecol.* 155:159–161, 1986.

Dengue

Centers for Disease Control, U.S. Dept. H.H.S. Dengue fever in U.S. military personnel—Republic of the Philippines. *Morbidity and Mortality Weekly Report* 34:495–502, 1985.

Centers for Disease Control, U.S. Dept. H.H.S. Dengue—The Americas, 1984. *Morbidity and Mortality Weekly Report.* 35:51–57, 1986.

Ventora, A., Ehrenkranz, N., and Rosenthal, D. Placental passage of antibodies to dengue virus in persons living in a region of hyper endemic dengue virus infection. *J. Infect. Dis.* 131:S62–S68, 1975.

Rabies

Burridge, M., et al. Intradermal immunization with human diploid cell rabies vaccine. *J.A.M.A.*, 248:1611–1614, 1982.

McCracken, G. Post-exposure rabies prophylaxis. *Pediatr. Infect. Dis.*, 3:S41, 1984.

Varner, M., McGuinness, G., and Galask, R. Rabies vaccination in pregnancy. *Am. J. Obstet. Gynecol.* 143:717–718, 1982.

Smallpox

Breman, J., and Arita, I. The confirmation and maintenance of smallpox eradication. *N. Engl. J. Med.* 303:1263–1273, 1980.
Feery, B. Adverse reactions after smallpox vaccination. *Med. J. Aust.* 6:180, 1977.
Nadeari, S. Smallpox vaccination during pregnancy. *Obstet. Gynecol.* 46:223–226, 1975.

II

Bacterial Infections

11 Gonorrhea

Gonorrhea is the most frequent sexually transmitted disease reported in the United States. The causative organism, *Neisseria gonorrhoeae,* is a gram-negative, kidney bean-shaped diplococcus first described by Neisser in 1879. Gonorrheal ophthalmia neonatorum, a major neonatal consequence of maternal infection, was a significant cause of blindness until the introduction of silver nitrate prophylaxis by Credé in 1881. Current problems for gonorrhea control include the spread of resistant strains and treatment of concurrent infections with other bacteria. (See Chap. 20, Chlamydia Infections.)

FREQUENCY

Approximately one million cases of gonorrhea are reported in the United States each year. Depending on the socioeconomic status of the population at risk and the frequency and number of sites screened, estimates of the frequency of gonorrheal infections in pregnancy have ranged from 0.5 to 7.0 percent. Although probably less prevalent in the first half of pregnancy than the second, asymptomatic colonization and symptomatic disease including salpingitis and disseminated sepsis can occur at any time during gestation. As the occurrence of gonorrhea in pregnancy becomes more widely recognized, associations with premature rupture of the membranes, chorioamnionitis, and neonatal sepsis are being reported with steadily increasing frequency.

In 1976 isolates of penicillinase-producing *N. gonorrhoeae* (PPNG) were first detected in the United States. The frequency of PPNG has increased steadily, with endemic foci in California, New York, and Florida to the point that several thousand cases are reported each year. In sexually transmitted disease clinics that have tested extensively for PPNG, frequencies as high as 30 to 50 percent have been reported. Strains of PPNG have been reported from all states. In 1983, an outbreak of infection due to chromosomally mediated resistant *N. gonorrhoeae* (CMRNG) was reported from North Carolina. Since the initial report of CMRNG, strains of gonococci with multiple drug resistance have also been reported from other parts of the United States, Africa, and Southeast Asia.

DIAGNOSIS

Mother

Pregnancy does not confer protection from gonorrhea, although 60 to 80 percent of all patients with gonorrhea in pregnancy are asymptomatic. In order to detect asymptomatic gonorrhea during pregnancy and minimize perinatal morbidity through prompt treatment, all pregnant women should have endocervical cultures for *N. gonorrhoeae* performed at the time of their first prenatal visit. Repeat cultures in the third trimester are warranted for patients at high risk of acquiring sexually transmitted disease during pregnancy.

Despite previous hypotheses that infection of the uterus might be prevented by the endocervical mucus plug, symptomatic gonorrhea during pregnancy does occur. In the first trimester, gonococcal salpingitis has been reported, although it is probably quite rare. Septic abortions have also been described. In the third trimester, cases of

Table 11-1. Diagnosis of Gonorrhea

Mother	Child
Clinical	
Most are asymptomatic Occasionally Pelvic peritonitis Premature rupture of membranes Chorioamnionitis Septic polyarthritis Septicemia with fever and rash Subacute bacterial endocarditis Meningitis	Unexplained sepsis Meningitis Fulminant purulent conjunctivitis Septic polyarthritis
Laboratory	
Genital swab—Gram's stain showing gram-negative diplococci or positive immunologic test (presumptive) Genital or blood cultures positive for *N. gonorrhoeae* Oral or rectal cultures as suggested by type of sexual exposure	Gram's stain of conjunctivitis shows many gram-negative diplococci Eye, blood, CSF cultures positive for gonorrhea

premature rupture of the membranes with chorioamnionitis have been associated with *N. gonorrhoeae*.

Disseminated infections causing arthritis, tenosynovitis, subacute bacterial endocarditis, meningitis, and septicemia also occur during pregnancy. A maculopapular rash, ultimately changing to necrotic pustules is not uncommon in disseminated disease. Of note is the frequent association between gonococcal arthritis and pregnancy. In most series, 40 percent of all cases of septic arthritis arise in gravidas, characteristically during the second or third trimester.

The differential diagnosis of gonococcal arthritis is facilitated by both clinical considerations and laboratory findings (Table 11-1). Reiter's syndrome and gout are infrequent diseases among women of childbearing age. Probably the most likely alternate diagnosis is acute rheumatic fever that is characterized by associated cardiac disease, an elevated antistreptolysin O titer, and usually dramatic response to salicylate therapy without antibiotics. Rheumatoid arthritis, on the other hand, is a symmetrical disease of small joints associated, in the majority of cases, with a positive serum rheumatoid factor.

Gonorrheal arthritis is a febrile illness frequently associated with asymmetric (unilateral) polyarthritis affecting medium and large joints. Monoarticular septic arthritis in a sexually active adult strongly suggests gonococcal arthritis. It responds dramatically to appropriate antibiotics. Genital cultures are frequently (though not invariably) positive for *N. gonorrhoeae*. When considering diagnostic arthrocentesis, the risk of iatrogenic joint infection should be weighed against the possible diagnostic benefit of successfully culturing the gonococcus from joint effusions. Gonorrheal arthritis should be seriously considered when the differential diagnosis of polyarthritis arises in pregnancy.

Laboratory diagnosis of gonorrhea requires isolation of the organism, usually on Thayer-Martin medium under CO_2 incubation. Although careful examination of gram-stained material correctly identifies 70 percent of all subsequently culture-verified cases, the implications of the diagnosis make it prudent to await the results of cultures before informing the patient about the nature of her infection. It is currently recommended that all isolates of *N. gonorrhoeae* be tested for penicillin resistance with agar containing 1 μg/ml of penicillin G.

A single endocervical culture detects 80 percent of all patients with gonorrhea, but it is appropriate to consider other possible sites of infection in pregnant women. In one survey of an antenatal clinic population, the oropharynx was the only positive culture site in 36 percent of all cases.

In addition to bacterial culturing, immunoassay techniques may be available in some institutions. Although these tests appear to be 97 percent specific, their sensitivity is less than 90 percent. Presently, such tests are not adequate alternatives to culture for screening during pregnancy.

Child

Gonococcal ophthalmia characteristically begins as a purulent conjunctivitis. If unrecognized and untreated, corneal ulcerations ensue, leading rapidly to corneal perforation and fibrosis with blindness. *Mima-Herellea* conjunctivitis can mimic the disease since this is also a purulent conjunctivitis caused by gram-negative diplococci. The clinical course of the latter infection is less fulminant, however, and cultural characteristics of the organisms differ. The differential diagnosis of conjunctivitis in neonates also includes chlamydia, currently the most common form of bacterial conjunctivitis of the newborn. (See Chap. 20, Chlamydia Infections.)

Neonatal gonococcal arthritis, presumably due to septicemia, occasionally occurs one to five weeks following delivery. The disease is characteristically a septic polyarthritis. Like its adult counterpart, it must be distinguished from acute rheumatic fever on clinical and laboratory grounds. Fetal sepsis in association with gonorrheal chorioamnionitis has also been reported. A possible association between premature rupture of the membranes and gonorrhea has been postulated as well.

PROGNOSIS IF UNTREATED

The prognosis for infants born to mothers with untreated gonorrhea is somewhat difficult to assess. Mothers in whom the diagnosis was missed at first and recognized in retrospect are often women who have received inadequate or no prenatal care. Their infants can be expected to suffer significant (10–20%) mortality due to stillbirth and prematurity.

MANAGEMENT

Mother and Child

Positive cultures for gonorrhea should be treated with amoxicillin or ampicillin by mouth, or ceftriaxone or aqueous procaine penicillin G, IM. All of these drugs except ceftriaxone should be accompanied by an oral bolus of probenecid. Since concomitant carriage of chlamydia may approach 30 percent and concomitant syphilis is not uncommon, a screening serology should be included at the time of initial therapy, and a test for chlamydia should be done or empiric erythromycin should be given for seven days (Table 11-2). Pregnant women who are allergic to the drugs noted above should be treated initially with spectinomycin 2.0 g, IM, followed by erythromycin.

Whether initial therapy should cover PPNG or CMRNG depends on the expected frequency of resistance in the population being treated. If coverage of resistance is desired for asymptomatic women, spectinomycin 2.0 g, IM, or ceftriaxone 250 mg, IM, followed by erythromycin as outlined in Table 11-2 is recommended. Follow-up culturing of the mother, review of serology, and treatment of contacts are essential to assure definitive therapy. Penicillinase-producing isolates of *N. gonorrhoeae* will be identified if positive cultures from treatment failures are tested for resistance to penicillin. The importance of culture follow-up to ensure adequacy of chemotherapy is emphasized. At least those patients with a positive culture earlier in pregnancy (and ideally, all high-risk patients) should be recultured at 36 weeks. Neonates infected with PPNG or CMRNG should be treated with cefotaxime or gentamicin in appropriate doses.

Women with pharyngeal gonococcal infection due to penicillin-sensitive strains should be treated with the standard penicillin and probenecid regimen (Table 11-2) since ampicillin, spectinomycin, and cefoxitin have been reported to have high clinical failure rates. Successful therapy of PPNG infection of the oropharynx during pregnancy has been reported by Soper and Merrill-Nach (1986). They used a daily single dose of nine tablets of trimethoprim/sulfamethoxazole (80 mg/400 mg) orally for five days; however, the safety and statistical effectiveness of this method remain to be established.

Patients with disseminated gonococcemia and septic arthritis should receive antibiotics as indicated by resistance patterns until there is remission of symptoms. Blood cultures should be obtained before initiation of treatment. Following abatement of symptoms, therapy may be adjusted as shown in Table 11-2. Intra-articular instillation of penicillin offers no substantive advantage in terms of therapeutic response and may precipitate a significant chemical synovitis. Sepsis in children should be treated with high-dose parenteral penicillin or ampicillin in divided doses for seven to ten days. Septic neonatal gonococcal arthritis may require longer therapy and, in infants and adults, consideration should be given to immobilization of affected joints by splinting as long as the patient remains symptomatic.

Neonatal ophthalmitis should prompt examination and therapy for both parents if they were previously unrecognized as infected. The infant should receive penicillin eye drops, in association with parenteral penicillin, for seven days. The potential gravity of this infection makes consultation by an ophthalmologist appropriate, and prompt evaluation by Gram's stain and culture of all neonatal conjunctivitis cannot be overemphasized.

PREVENTION

The increasing frequency with which asymptomatic gonorrheal infection occurs in women makes screening appropriate in the prenatal clinic. Promiscuity and low socioeconomic status, previously useful markers for populations at risk, should be expanded to include more contemporary covariants such as adolescent and drug-dependent mothers. Contemporary sexual mores dictate a more thorough examination of all potential sites of infection in such women.

Table 11-2. Treatment and Follow-up of Gonorrhea

Mother	Child
Treatment	
Asymptomatic Genital Gonorrhea Amoxicillin 3.0 g, PO, or Ampicillin 3.5 g, PO, or Ceftriaxone 250 mg., IM, or Aqueous procaine penicillin G 4.8 million U IM (amoxicillin, ampicillin, and penicillin regimens are accompanied by probenecid 1.0 g PO) PLUS Erythromycin base 500 mg, PO qid × 7 days, or Erythromycin ethylsuccinate 800 mg, PO qid × 7 days	*Asymptomatic infant of untreated mother* Aqueous crystalline penicillin G 50,000 U IV or IM for full-term neonates. Decrease dose for low birthweight infants
Disseminated Gonococcal Infection Aqueous crystalline penicillin G 10 million U IV per day × 3 days followed by amoxicillin or ampicillin 500 mg PO qid × 7 days of therapy, or Amoxicillin 3.0 g or ampicillin 3.5 g each with probenecid 1.0 g PO followed by amoxicillin or ampicillin 500 mg PO qid × 7 days, or Cefoxitin 1.0 g IV qid × 7 days, or Cefotaxime 500 mg IV qid × 7 days, or Ceftriaxone 1.0 g IV once daily × 7 days PLUS Erythromycin, as above	Penicillin 75,000–100,000 U IV in divided doses or Ampicillin 50 mg/kg/day IV or IM in divided doses for 7–10 days
Gonococcal Ophthalmia Aqueous penicillin G 10 million U IV daily × 5 days Cefoxitin 1.0 g IV × 5 days, or Cefotaxime 500 mg IV qid × 5 days, or Ceftriaxone 1.0 g IM daily × 5 days	Aqueous crystalline penicillin G 100,000 U/kg/day IV in 4 divided doses × 7 days
Follow-up	
Repeat cultures 7–14 days following therapy and prior to delivery*	Cultures as appropriate

*Serologic testing for syphilis and chlamydia should be part of the management of pregnant women with gonorrhea.

Despite the apparent efficacy of routine eye prophylaxis in preventing ophthalmitis in neonates, a few treatment failures can be anticipated despite such measures. These failures will be minimized provided the solution is applied directly to the conjunctival sac within one hour of birth and care is taken to avoid flushing the medication out of the eye prematurely. The traditional silver nitrate eye prophylaxis is still effective for all strains of gonococcus; however, erythromycin eye prophylaxis is now being widely used to attempt to provide prophylaxis for chlamydia in addition to *N. gonorrhoeae*.

Finally, by relaying information about antepartum gonorrheal treatment and follow-up to their pediatric colleagues, obstetricians can aid considerably in neonatal surveillance for potential complications. Ophthalmic prophylaxis may not control circumstances when gonococcal attachment and engulfment has already occurred, further underscoring the importance of careful neonatal follow-up.

QUESTIONS AND ANSWERS

1. *How can false-negatives be minimized in screening for gonorrhea during pregnancy?*

   Some false-negatives may result from failure to culture all potential sites of infection and thus represent errors in sampling. Moreover, cervical cultures obtained from women with gonorrhea frequently include a substantial number of other aerobic and anaerobic organisms. Unless special care is exercised, overgrowth by such bacteria can make recovery of the fastidious gonococcus impossible. Ideally, direct inoculation of specimens on modified Thayer-Martin medium with 10% CO_2 atmosphere should be accomplished in the examination room. Alternatively, Martin-Lester transport medium may be employed, provided that it is incubated before transport. In the unlikely event that logistics prevent screening of patients using either method, consideration can be given to using a non-nutritive transport medium. Modified Stuart medium with charcoal has been successfully used to recover *N. gonorrhoeae* provided that specimens are transported promptly to the laboratory for plating—in all instances within 24 hours. Charcoal absorbs and neutralizes certain fatty acids found in plain agar, which are inhibitory to gonococcal growth. Thayer-Martin culture plates or Martin-Lester transport medium are preferable to Stuart medium for *N. gonorrhoeae* in all cases.

2. *What therapy is appropriate for a woman with a history of penicillin allergy who has disseminated gonococcemia in the second trimester of pregnancy?*

   Significant gonococcal infections in the penicillin-allergic gravida present difficult therapeutic decisions. Alternative drug regimens such as tetracycline are associated with unacceptable fetal complications of therapy. Erythromycin might be considered as an alternative but it may not adequately treat infection in the fetal compartment.

   Consideration might first be given to skin testing and historical review of the nature of the drug reaction to document or refute penicillin sensitivity. Spectinomycin and kanamycin have been used for uncomplicated salpingitis, but there is little clinical experience with either in disseminated gonococcal disease. Moreover, the safety of spectinomycin in pregnancy has not been established.

   Cephalothin derivatives are reported to be associated with 10 percent incidence of cross-sensitivity in penicillin-allergic patients. Cefoxitin, cefotaxime, or ceftriaxone are highly effective and include coverage of PPNG strains. If penicillin therapy is believed to be necessary despite the allergy, as when the patient has concomitant syphilis, intravenous penicillin desensitization and treatment may be attempted during pregnancy (Ziaya et al., 1986).

SELECTED READINGS

Centers for Disease Control, U.S. Dept. H.H.S. 1985 STD treatment guidelines. *Morbidity and Mortality Weekly Report* 34(4S):81S–86S, 1985.

Faruki, H., et al. A community-based outbreak of infection with penicillin-resistant *Neisseria gonorrhoeae* not producing penicillinase (chromosomally mediated resistance). *N. Engl. J. Med.* 313:607–611, 1985.

Holmes, K., Counts, G., and Beaty, H. Disseminated gonococcal infection. *Ann. Intern. Med.* 74:979–993, 1971.

Pierog, S., et al. Gonococcal ophthalmia neonatorum. *Am. J. Obstet. Gynecol.* 122:589–592, 1975.

Rice, R., and Thompson, S. Treatment of uncomplicated infections due to *Neisseria gonorrhoeae:* A review of clinical efficacy and in vitro susceptibility studies from 1982 through 1985. *J.A.M.A.* 255:1739–1746, 1986.

Sarrel, P., and Pruett, K. Symptomatic gonorrhea during pregnancy. *Obstet. Gynecol.* 32:670–673, 1968.

Soper, D., and Merrill-Nach, S. Successful therapy of penicillinase-producing *Neisseria gonorrhoeae* pharyngeal infection during pregnancy. *Obstet. Gynecol.* 68:290–291, 1986.

Ziaya, P., et al. Intravenous penicillin desensitization and treatment during pregnancy. *J.A.M.A.* 256:2561–2562, 1986.

12 Syphilis

While congenital syphilis is the most severe form of syphilitic disease, it can be prevented or treated in utero if the mother receives optimal prenatal diagnosis and antimicrobial therapy. In the 17th century, the infection of infants with syphilis became generally known, although infection in utero was not widely recognized. In 1767, John Hunter developed syphilis following self-inoculation, but he did not distinguish between syphilis and gonorrhea. It is now recognized that syphilis is due to the spirochete *Treponema pallidum.*

FREQUENCY

The frequency of syphilis in adults varies widely according to sexual exposure of the individuals concerned. Incidence is very low in married women with faithful spouses, while it is highest among prostitutes. The risk of contracting syphilis by sexual contact with a partner having a primary or secondary infection appears to be about 50 percent. Approximately 8000 cases of primary and secondary syphilis in women are reported in the United States annually. More than 80 percent of these women are of reproductive age, and thereby at risk of having a child with congenital syphilis. Approximately 160 cases of congenital syphilis are reported in the United States each year. Women giving birth to these children generally have had inadequate prenatal care.

The risk for the child is present throughout pregnancy. Previously intrauterine syphilis was considered impossible before the middle of gestation; however, Harter and Benirschke (1976) have shown that early pregnancies can be infected as well. It is believed that the degree of risk for infection of the fetus bears some relationship to the quantity of spirochetes circulating in the maternal bloodstream. Spirochetemia is expected to be more common during primary or secondary syphilis than during latent syphilis; therefore, it is expected that women with acute syphilis during pregnancy would be more likely to produce a baby with congenital syphilis than individuals who had untreated latent syphilis of several years' duration. In 1952, Fiumara and associates reported that when a pregnant woman had primary or secondary syphilis, her child had a 50 percent probability of having congenital syphilis, while the risk of congenital syphilis decreased to 40 percent in children of mothers with early latent disease, and further decreased to 10 percent in children of mothers with late syphilis.

DIAGNOSIS

Mother

The diagnosis of syphilis may be based on a combination of physical findings, epidemiology, and laboratory tests (Table 12-1). The physical findings of early infection include the oft-mentioned but seldom seen chancre of primary syphilis and the skin rash of secondary syphilis. *T. pallidum* can be seen on darkfield examination of wet smears for such lesions. Physical findings of late syphilis include well-known pathologic findings of every organ system. Clinical and histologic findings of late syphilis may be sufficient to establish the diagnosis regardless of serologic testing.

Table 12-1. Diagnosis of Syphilis

Mother	Child
Epidemiology	
Sexual contact with known syphilitic partner	Born of syphilitic mother. If maternal infection occurred late in pregnancy, child may be seronegative, yet still infected
Physical findings	
Early syphilis Primary lesion: chancre, a painless papule that becomes an ulcer. This lesion depends on inoculum size and immunity and may vary in appearance Secondary lesion: disseminated lymphadenopathy and rash. Can include palms and soles, maculopapular. Each lesion can be up to 10 mm diameter and can become pustular. Enlarged papules can form condylomalata. Mucosal erosions are common. Lesions of hair follicles can produce alopecia. Eye lesions include iritis and chorioretinitis Latent syphilis Normal physical exam Late syphilis Gummas, neurosyphilis, cardiovascular changes *rarely* seen in pregnant women	Early congenital syphilis Most are asymptomatic. No chancres seen. In symptomatic, live-born children, maculopapular rash that may progress to desquamation or bullae, mucous patches, rhinitis, hepatosplenomegaly, jaundice, lymphadenopathy, edema, deformed nails, alopecia, chorioretinitis, iritis, fever, pseudoparalysis
Laboratory	
Darkfield exam Can be positive from primary or secondary lesions Nonspecific serologic tests (RPR, VDRL) False-positive may occur during pregnancy with other concurrent infectious disease, narcotic abuse, or autoimmune disease. False-negative common in primary, latent, and late syphilis Specific serologic tests (FTA-ABS, MHA-TP, TPI) Not used for screening Spinal fluid (CSF) Pleocytosis, elevated protein, positive CSF VDRL indicate neurosyphilis Diagnostic value of CSF FTA-ABS unknown General Elevated SGOT + alkaline phosphate if syphilitic hepatitis is present; proteinura or hematuria if renal syphilis is present	From mucocutaneous lesions Can be false-positive owing to passive transfer of IgG antibody from mother IgM FTA-ABS test may be useful, if available Pleocytosis, elevated protein, and positive CSF VDRL indicate congenital neurosyphilis Radiological Osteochondritis at joints of extremities; periostitis of long bones and skull, widened, irregular, and sometimes separated epiphyses

Women who are diagnosed as having syphilis while pregnant are usually asymptomatic. Diagnosis may be strongly suspected based on a history of intimate contact with persons known to be syphilitic. Usually, the diagnosis is based on serologic testing, done either as routine screening or to follow up clinical suspicion.

The serologic tests used are nonspecific tests for reagin-type antibodies, or specific antitreponemal antibody tests. Nonspecific antibody tests for syphilis in use today include the VDRL, the Kolmer test, and the rapid plasma reagin (RPR) test. The specific treponemal antibody tests most commonly used are the fluorescent treponemal antibody absorption test (FTA-ABS) and the microhemagglutination test for syphilis (MHA-TP). The *Treponema pallidum* immobilization (TPI) test is also a specific antibody test that is less commonly used but has for many years been the ultimate standard for diagnosis. Immunofluorescence and immunoperoxidase methods have been adapted for the identification of *T. pallidum* in tissue, as may be necessary from an abortus specimen.

It is recommended that all pregnant women have a serologic test performed for syphilis at the time of the first prenatal visit, and women who are at risk for acquiring a sexually transmitted disease should be screened again in the third trimester.

The usual sequence for serologic testing during pregnancy begins with the RPR. If the RPR is positive, usually a quantitative VDRL test is performed automatically. Then, the clinician may order the FTA-ABS test if the diagnosis of syphilis has not been made previously. If all tests are positive, then the diagnosis of syphilis is established. Neither the FTA-ABS test nor the TPI test is efficient for large-scale screening measures, since they require a great amount of laboratory technician time and concentration to be performed properly.

False-positive reactions can occur with all of these tests but are uncommon with the specific antitreponemal tests. Common causes of a false-positive nontreponemal test include other infectious diseases, narcotics abuse, autoimmune diseases, and possibly pregnancy itself. False-positive reactions are most often only weak or borderline reactions. Frequently, false-positive tests are qualitatively atypical laboratory reactions that can be detected and reported by an alert technician performing the test. To maximize treatment of the fetus at risk, it is customary to consider a positive FTA-ABS or MHA-TP test to be truly positive rather than falsely positive in a pregnant woman.

Whether every woman who is asymptomatic but has positive serologic diagnosis of syphilis should then have a spinal tap done during the pregnancy is controversial. The benefits of a spinal tap done during the pregnancy in virtually all cases outweigh the possible risks. Spinal tap allows the detection of asymptomatic neurosyphilis, its proper treatment, and follow-up. By making the diagnosis more specific, the prognosis can be outlined with greater surety. Treatment also depends on the diagnosis that was made. The physician is obliged to treat for asymptomatic neurosyphilis if a spinal puncture has not been performed. The current treatment recommendations for asymptomatic neurosyphilis require a series of injections. Patient compliance and return for continuation of a series of injections is difficult in many settings, especially where one is dealing with a clinic group in which return visits seem to decrease with the increasing number of injections.

The diagnosis of reinfection or persistence of active syphilis can be made in a patient previously known to have had syphilis by following the titer of the VDRL test. A rising titer would indicate a need for further diagnostic measures such as spinal tap and appropriate treatment.

Following primary infection, 25 percent of untreated or inadequately treated women develop a secondary form of the disease within four years. Without treatment, ultimately a minimum of 10 percent of patients with primary or secondary syphilis develop cardiovascular syphilis, and 16 percent develop neurosyphilis. These are probably the minimal estimates of risk. Inclusion of asymptomatic persons found at autopsy to have cardiovascular disease or neurosyphilis would increase this estimate. If untreated, ultimately, 10 percent of syphilis patients will die from this disease.

Child

Congenital neurosyphilis may be diagnosed readily in the florid case where a hydropic fetus and placenta are delivered and laboratory studies show the typical features of the disease. Such infected offspring were far more common before the antibiotic era. Now it is more common for the infected newborn to be asymptomatic at birth but to have a positive nonspecific test for syphilis in the cord blood. The problem is to decide whether this is merely IgG antibody passively transferred from the mother or whether it is IgM antibody that represents a true fetal infection. An IgM FTA-ABS test has been developed; however, there are problems with the test related to separating the IgM from the IgG. Anyone who uses such a test should be careful to know what the quality of separation is. If this separation is performed too vigorously, there can be false-negative tests due to loss of IgM that is truly present. In addition, false-positive tests are sometimes due to inclusion of a small amount of IgG with the presumed IgM fraction. Fetal rheumatoid factor (fetal IgM against maternal IgG) will also cause a false-positive IgM FTA-ABS test. When congenital syphilis is suspected, a spinal tap should be performed. Laboratory examination of a newborn's cerebrospinal fluid (CSF) may indicate that asymptomatic neurosyphilis is present. When the spinal fluid VDRL is positive, the diagnosis of asymptomatic congenital neurosyphilis is made. Microscopic examination of the CSF may show leukocytes and protein; however, this should be considered a relatively nonspecific finding. Examination of normal CSF following a routine delivery can show 20–35 leukocytes/mm^3 and 100–150 mg/100 ml protein.

Incompletely treated early congenital syphilis will progress to the classic manifestations of late congenital syphilis. By 10 to 13 years of age, an affected child may have developed gummas as well as neural, bony, dental, and cardiovascular stigmata of advanced syphilis.

MANAGEMENT

Mother

All gravidas with positive, specific tests for syphilis should be treated unless there is good evidence of adequate prior treatment and no suspicion that reinfection has occurred. In practice, it is usually better to retreat than omit therapy when previous therapy is unknown.

Penicillin is the best treatment available for syphilis. The secondary drugs that have been studied are tetracycline and erythromycin. It is recommended that tetracycline not be used during pregnancy for the treatment of syphilis. Tetracycline can be hepatotoxic for the pregnant woman and can be deposited in the teeth and bones of the child. Erythromycin when used properly has satisfactory results for the mother; although due to very minimal placental transfer of this drug, it is usually necessary to give the baby further treatment after birth to assure adequate care. For women with a history of penicillin allergy, an alternative management plan that would provide satisfactory treatment for both mother and fetus includes allergy testing, penicillin desensitization, and continuous intravenous infusion of aqueous penicillin G (25,000 U/hr) for 8 days (Ziaya et al., 1986).

The antibiotic treatment schedules for syphilis are given in Table 12-2. The drug dosages given for the treatment of syphilis are the minimum amounts considered to be effective for the cure of the disease. A larger dose can be given if it is deemed proper in the clinical judgment of the doctor managing the patient. Some experts have recommended that the treatment of early syphilis include a repeat of the initial penicillin treatment after one week. The proposed treatment regimens for neurosyphilis have not been thoroughly studied and may have a failure rate of approximately 10 percent. Neurosyphilis patients should be managed in consultation with an expert. Given adequate treatment, the prognosis for the mother should be excellent.

Other drugs including ampicillin, cephalosporins, streptomycin, and chloramphenicol have been used in the treatment of syphilis. However, such drugs have somewhat less efficacy than that of penicillin, and recommendations regarding the use of these drugs cannot be made. The principle of the treatment of syphilis with penicillin is to maintain a blood antibiotic level over a long period of time to cover properly the long (>30 hr) replication time of the organism. Thus, since *T. pallidum* remains exquisitely sensitive to low doses of penicillin, benzathine penicillin has been the form used and proved in practice through the years.

Gravidas who have been treated for early syphilis should be followed with monthly nontreponemal serologic tests for syphilis. Treatment should be repeated if there is either a 4-fold increase in titer or if a 4-fold decrease in titer does not occur during a three-month period (Centers for Disease Control, 1985). Syphilis treated within six months of onset of infection results in seroreversion to a negative reaginic test in virtually all cases within 12 months; however, lifelong reaginic seropositivity may occur when syphilis has been present for a long time (approximately 1 year or more) prior to treatment. Following development of a positive FTA-ABS or MHA-TP test, these specific treponemal tests remain positive for life and, thus, are not useful in the clinical follow-up of women known to have had syphilis.

Child

The neonatologist is faced with a dilemma when told that an asymptomatic baby has a positive nonspecific cord blood test for syphilis. If all babies with a positive serology were treated vigorously with a course of penicillin, then a great number of babies would be overtreated since, in many cases, the pediatrician would be treating an infant with passive transfer of antibody and not one with true congenital disease.

A thorough maternal history documented by the obstetrician enables the pediatrician to tailor the treatment as appropriate. When the obstetrician can provide only a weak or vague history of the

Table 12-2. Management of Syphilis*

Mother	Child
Duration of syphilis *less* than one year (primary, secondary, or latent): Benzathine penicillin G, 2.4 million U, IM at one session (If allergic to penicillin; erythromycin-stearate, ethylsuccinate, or base—500 mg PO qid for 15 days) Duration of syphilis *more* than one year (latent, cardiovascular, late benign, except neurosyphilis): Benzathine penicillin G, 7.2 million U total given IM as 2.4 million U at weekly intervals (If allergic to penicillin: erythromycin-stearate, ethylsuccinate, or base—500 mg PO qid for 30 days) Neurosyphilis Aqueous crystalline penicillin G 12–24 million U IV/day (in divided doses every 4 hrs) for 10 days, followed by benzathine penicillin G 2.4 million U IM weekly for 3 doses or Aqueous procaine penicillin G 2.4 million U IM daily plus probenecid 500 mg PO qid, both for 10 days, followed by benzathine penicillin 2.4 million U IM weekly for 3 doses or Benzathine penicillin G 2.4 million U IM weekly for 3 doses N.B. Avoid treatment with tetracycline during pregnancy	Skin contact isolation for first 24 hours of treatment is advised for newborn with congenital syphilis and lesions of skin or mucous membranes Any child suspected of having congenital syphilis should have a CSF exam before treatment Newborns with abnormal CSF Aqueous crystalline penicillin G, 50,000 U/kg IM or IV daily in two divided doses for a minimum of 10 days or Aqueous procaine penicillin G, 50,000 U/kg IM daily for a minimum of 10 days Newborns with normal CSF: Benzathine penicillin G, 50,000 U/kg IM in a single dose If the infant's mother was adequately treated with penicillin during pregnancy, or known to be sero-fast, treatment can be withheld from the infant, provided there is adequate follow-up serologic testing of the infant until the RPR or VDRL has become negative All individuals treated for syphilis should have follow-up serologic testing. Retreatment should be considered when (1) clinical signs or symptoms persist; (2) there is a sustained 4-fold increase in titer of nontreponemal test; (3) an initially high-titer nontreponemal test fails to show a 4-fold decrease in one year Examination should be performed before treatment

*Adapted from Centers for Disease Control, *Morbidity and Mortality Weekly Report.* 34(4S):94S–99S, 1985.

duration of the disease and prior treatment, then it is incumbent upon the pediatrician to give the child the full course of treatment. If the quantitative VDRL from the newborn is higher than the simultaneous test from the mother, or if the baby's IgM FTA-ABS test is positive, then the baby should be treated. Follow-up for the child with a positive VDRL remains important to ensure that treatment has been adequate. A rising titer is a sign of continued activity of the disease and an indication for further treatment.

In cases where treatment of the mother during pregnancy was with erythromycin only, it is particularly important either to treat the child at birth or follow the child's titer monthly until the titer is zero. A persistent or rising titer in such cases indicates that treatment should be started.

PREVENTION

After the discovery of penicillin, it was hoped that syphilis would be eliminated. *T. pallidum* has remained extremely sensitive to the drug. However, the power of promiscuity plus inaccurate diagnosis and management remain sufficient to ensure that the disease remains a problem.

The number of congenitally syphilitic infants will be minimized if physicians caring for pregnant women perform serologic testing for syphilis at the first antenatal visit and again in the third trimester. It is the responsibility of the obstetrician to (1) distinguish the patient with a false-positive nonspecific test from the true syphilitic, (2) ensure adequate treatment during pregnancy, and (3) ensure adequate communication of diagnosis and treatment to the physician who will care for the newborn.

The physician responsible for a newborn with a positive cord blood serologic test for syphilis should be certain that adequate therapy has been given and that adequate follow-up will be obtained. The risk of late syphilis following inadequate therapy for infants is sufficient to justify penicillin treatment of all newborns in whom the diagnosis cannot be excluded or in whom follow-up is expected to be poor.

QUESTIONS AND ANSWERS

1. *Can syphilis be acquired from doorknobs and toilet seats?*

   Seldom, if ever. When a patient suggests such transmission, the physician should adamantly, yet tactfully, pursue establishing and treating the source of intimate personal contact. Fluid from an infectious lesion must make contact with the recipient's area of inoculation. A chancre will develop at the inoculation site. It is well to remember that skin lesions of secondary syphilis are infectious. Blood on contaminated injection equipment may be the source of syphilis transmission among drug users.

2. *Does the treatment of gonorrhea cure syphilis?*

   No, unless the syphilis is incubating (not yet seropositive) or the treatment is prolonged (as in the treatment of gonococcal salpingitis).

3. *Should a pregnant woman with syphilis be given different theapy from a nonpregnant woman?*

   Tetracycline should not be used during pregnancy. While a higher dosage of penicillin has been recommended by some for treating pregnant women, such treatment has not been shown to be necessary. The treatment schedule for penicillin shows the minimum dosage that usually is effective (Table 11-2). More penicillin can be given if desired, particularly if neurosyphilis has been diagnosed, in an effort to minimize the possibility that *T. pallidum* may persist if inadequately treated across the blood-brain barrier.

SELECTED READINGS

Centers for Disease Control, U.S. Dept. H.H.S. 1985 standard treatment guidelines. *Morbidity and Mortality Weekly Report* 34(4S):94S–99S, 1985.

Ducas, J. and Robson, H. Cerebrospinal fluid levels during therapy for latent syphilis. *J.A.M.A.* 246:2583–2584, 1981.

Fiumara, N., et al. The incidence of prenatal syphilis at the Boston City Hospital. *N. Engl. J. Med.* 247:48–54, 1952.

Guinan, M. Treatment of primary and secondary syphilis: Defining failure at three- and six-month followup. *J.A.M.A.* 257:340–359, 1987.

Harter, C., and Benirschke, K. Fetal syphilis in the first trimester. *Am. J. Obstet. Gynecol.* 124:705–711, 1976.

Mascola, L., et al. Congenital syphilis: Why is it still occurring? *J.A.M.A.* 252:1719–1722, 1984.

McCracken, G., and Kaplan, J. Penicillin treatment for congenital syphilis: A critical re-appraisal. *J.A.M.A.* 228:855–858, 1974.

Ziaya, P., et al. Intravenous penicillin desensitization and treatment during pregnancy. *J.A.M.A.* 256:2561–2562, 1986.

13

Group B Streptococcal Infections

Infectious syndromes due to streptococci are significant sources of perinatal morbidity and mortality. Using the serologic classification suggested by Lancefield in 1933, group A streptococci have been recognized as a cause of fatal puerperal sepsis. Group B streptococci have been long known in veterinary medicine as a cause of bovine mastitis. Human puerperal endometritis caused by group B streptococci is generally less severe than that caused by group A organisms. Group B streptococci have become recognized as a prominent cause of newborn sepsis and meningitis. (Consideration of disease due to other streptococci is contained in Chap. 15, Chorioamnionitis, and 16, Neonatal Sepsis.)

FREQUENCY

Asymptomatic colonization with group B streptococci occurs in approximately 15 to 30 percent of pregnant women. The colonization rate shows geographic variability even when optimal culture techniques have been used. When the babies born to women known to have positive vaginal cultures for group B streptococci have been cultured, the transmission rate from mother to baby at birth has been approximately 50 to 75 percent.

The proven colonization rate has been far higher than the attack rate for newborn infection. The overall attack rate for early-onset neonatal sepsis due to group B streptococci has been 2 to 3 per 1000 live births. The estimated attack rate for late-onset neonatal infection has been 0.5 to 1.0 per 1000 live births. The attack rate for premature infants increases dramatically, to approximately 7 percent for babies weighing less than 1000 g at birth.

The rate of symptomatic maternal infection due to group B streptococci is also a fraction of the colonization rate. The rate of postpartum fever reported by Baker and associates (1975) was 22 percent in women colonized during the second trimester and 4 percent in controls. As with other bacterial causes of puerperal infection, the attack rate for disease due to group B streptococci is expected to increase with inoculum size, operative delivery, and duration of amniorrhexis. (See Chap. 15, Chorioamnionitis.) Also, maternal urinary tract infection can be due to the group B streptococci. Various studies have shown that group B streptococci cause 1 to 5 percent of urinary tract infections.

DIAGNOSIS

Mother

Asymptomatic genitourinary or gastrointestinal colonization with group B streptococci can be diagnosed by traditional culture methods or by rapid tests that use growth enhancement methods or immunologic methods to detect specific bacterial antigens. In studies that have screened asymptomatic women, the yield of positive cultures has varied with the techniques used. The highest yield of group B streptococci is found when a selective medium containing Todd-

Hewitt broth, sheep blood, nalidixic acid, and gentamicin is used so that streptococci are not masked by overgrowth of other bacteria (Baker, et al., 1973). When selective media are not used, 50 percent of genital cultures may be falsely negative for group B streptococci.

In the laboratory, the group B streptococci are usually identified by the following characteristics:

1. Beta hemolysis (except that 2–5 percent are nonhemolytic)
2. Bacitracin resistance (except that 5 percent are susceptible)
3. Hippurate hydrolysis (few exceptions)
4. Inability to hydrolyze esculin in 40 percent bile
5. Enhancement of staphylococcal beta hemolysis (CAMP test)

Less commonly, precipitin testing may be done on pure cultures. Latex fixation and immunofluorescence tests have been developed that can rapidly identify both hemolytic and nonhemolytic group B streptococci.

Symptomatic maternal genitourinary tract infection due to the group B streptococci may be associated with a range of manifestations including fever, chills, uterine tenderness, dysuria, urgency, and pyuria. None of these manifestations is specific for disease due to group B streptococci. The diagnoses of chorioamnionitis, puerperal sepsis, endometritis, cystitis, pyelonephritis, and wound infection can be supported by positive cultures for group B or other streptococci. (See Chap. 14, Urinary Tract Infections, and Chap. 15, Chorioamnionitis.)

Child

The great majority of colonized newborns are asymptomatic. Techniques for identifying group B streptococci in newborns are the same as for adults. To maximize detection of colonization, selective media should be used, and sampling should include the umbilicus, throat, external auditory canal, and rectum. Symptomatic infections in neonates have been divided into two syndromes (Table 13-1).

Early-Onset Syndrome

This syndrome appears within the first week of life and usually within the first two days. The majority of symptomatic newborns are of low birth weight. In its fulminant form, the early-onset syndrome appears as septic shock accompanied by respiratory distress leading to death within several hours despite appropriate antibiotic treatment. The fatality rate exceeds 50 percent. When less severe, the main clinical features of this syndrome may be almost indistinguishable from the respiratory distress syndrome. There is a strong association between early onset infection and maternal conditions such as premature amniorrhexis and chorioamnionitis, which are associated with bacterial colonization of the uterine cavity before birth; however, early-onset syndrome also can develop in term infants with no maternal risk factors. Meningitis may be present in approximately 30 percent of early-onset infections.

None of the clinical manifestations is sufficient to diagnose group B streptococcal disease in the absence of a positive laboratory test; however, the diagnosis may be suggested by the predominance of gram-positive cocci in the amniotic fluid or gastric aspirate or by a positive rapid assay. Decreased lung compliance may help the clinician to distinguish pneumonitis due to group B streptococci from idiopathic respiratory distress syndrome.

Table 13-1. Diagnosis of Group B Streptococcal Infection

Mother	Child
Clinical	
Most asymptomatic	Most asymptomatic
Evidence of symptomatic infection: Fever and chills Low abdominal pain, uterine tenderness Dysuria, urgency, costovertebral angle pain, tenderness Wound erythema, induration, purulent drainage	Early-onset syndrome Onset before one week old Apnea (most common) Pneumonia Shock Meningitis (30%) Late-onset syndrome Onset after one week old Meningitis (most common) Localized infection may be found in any of the following: eyes, sinuses, joints, bones, skin, ears, lungs
Laboratory	
Positive culture Rapid assay may use growth enhancement or immunologic methods	Specific diagnosis depends on positive culture of blood or cerebrospinal fluid. Rapid assay may permit presumptive diagnosis without delay Nonspecific findings Early-onset syndrome Chest x-ray consistent with RDS or pneumonia Gastric aspirate showing cocci and leukocytes Late-onset syndrome Spinal fluid leukocytosis and increased protein content

Late-Onset Syndrome

This syndrome usually appears after the first week of life. The majority of these infants have meningitis as a prominent clinical manifestation. Although the mortality is lower than that following early-onset infection, up to 50 percent of babies who have meningitis show subsequent neurologic defects. Late-onset infection may include localized infection in the middle ears, sinuses, conjunctiva, breasts, lungs, bones, joints, and skin. These manifestations are found much less often than meningitis.

Meningitis appears to be significantly related to the serotype of group B streptococci. There are five serotypes of group B streptococci (Ia, Ib, Ic, II, III), according to a classification scheme based on capsular polysaccharide antigens. Although serotyping of group B streptococci is not done by clinical laboratories, research studies have shown that more than 80 percent of early-onset infections in which meningitis was present were due to type III organisms. More than 95 percent of all late-onset infections in which meningitis is usually present are due to type III group B streptococci. These findings are in contrast to the more even distribution of the various serotypes among

Table 13-2. Management of Symptomatic Group B Streptococcal Infection

Mother	Child
Penicillin (drug of choice)	
Intravenous aqueous crystalline penicillin G, up to 20 million U daily in divided doses depending on severity of disease. Minimum dose should be 1 million U intravenously every six hours	Aqueous penicillin G—150,000–200,000 U/kg IV daily in 4 divided doses, when meningitis is documented not present. Increase dosage to 250,000–400,000 U/kg/day in 4–6 divided doses when meningitis is present
Ampicillin or cephalothin	**Ampicillin**
2 g IV loading dose, then 1 g IV every 4–6 hours depending on severity of illness	200 mg/kg/day IM or IV in 4–6 divided doses, when meningitis is not present. Increase dosage to 300 mg/kg/day in 4–6 doses IV when meningitis is present
Erythromycin	
250 mg PO every six hours. Dose may be doubled for more severe infections 15–20 mg/kg/day continuous IV infusion	NOT recommended

asymptomatic mothers (type Ia + Ib + Ic~⅓, type II~⅓, type III ~⅓).

While early-onset infection has been related to transmission from the mother's genital tract during parturition, that route of infection transmission seems to occur less often in late-onset disease. Nosocomial transmission of group B streptococci can occur in the newborn nursery by cross-colonization from other infants. Transmission probably occurs by direct contact (e.g., from colonized nursery staff) rather than through the respiratory portal. Other colonized infants appear to acquire group B streptococci by community contact after discharge from the hospital.

MANAGEMENT

For symptomatic infection due to group B streptococci, penicillin is the drug of choice if the infecting organism has been identified before starting treatment (Table 13-2). This is not usual; rather, a broader-spectrum antibiotic such as ampicillin is used as the initial drug for empirically treating the mother or the newborn. (See Chaps. 15, 16, Chorioamnionitis, Neonatal Sepsis.) The usual minimum inhibitory concentration (MIC) of penicillin G reported for group B streptococci is 0.02 μg/ml; however, some strains have been shown to have MIC as high as 0.6 μg/ml.

A 1 to 2 μg/ml concentration of penicillin may be expected in the neonate's spinal fluid during high-dose intravenous treatment. Therefore, in the treatment of newborn meningitis, it is recommended that penicillin G be maintained at 250,000 to 400,000 U/kg/day IV to achieve sufficient penicillin concentration in the cerebrospinal fluid to eradicate all streptococci. Treatment should be continued for 10 to 14 days.

Although ampicillin and penicillin both cross the placenta from maternal blood to fetal blood and amniotic fluid, there is no evidence that human babies can be treated and cured of congenital streptococcal infection by antepartum antimicrobial therapy alone. If maternal symptoms of amniotic fluid infection are present before delivery, antimicrobial therapy is indicated before birth. (See Chap. 15, Chorioamnionitis.) If the amniotic fluid is known to be colonized with group B streptococci, then antepartum and intrapartum antimicrobial therapy is advised even for asymptomatic women.

The risk of severe early-onset infection manifested in the baby at birth needs to be weighed against the risk of masking neonatal infection that could become symptomatic later. A common approach to this dilemma when a specific pathogen has not been identified is to withhold antibiotic treatment of the minimally symptomatic mother until immediately after delivery. This may be particularly appropriate when cesarean section is performed on a woman with (1) only mild pyrexia or (2) no pyrexia, but whose amniotic fluid smear showed bacteria and neutrophils.

PREVENTION

Although a variety of protocols for preventing perinatal infection due to group B streptococci have been proposed, there is no consensus regarding the best prevention strategy. Antepartum prophylactic treatment of women with positive vaginal cultures for group B streptococci has not been completely effective owing in part to venereal transmission of the organism. Further, the high ratio of maternal colonization to neonatal infection would require treatment of about 100 pregnant women for each possible case of early onset infection.

Although antepartum prophylaxis may not eliminate colonization from asymptomatic women, intrapartum ampicillin given intravenously has been shown to be highly effective in preventing mother-to-baby transmission and neonatal infection. This approach may be logically extended to instances with premature labor, premature amniorrhexis, or prolonged amniorrhexis in which there is proven or assumed colonization with group B streptococci. Boyer and Gotoff (1986) have suggested that screening cultures be done at 26 to 28 weeks' gestation so that women with positive cultures may be treated with intravenous ampicillin at the time of preterm labor or if there were prolonged amniorrhexis. Difficulties with this approach include the requirement for comprehensive screening, rapid reporting of results, and the phenomenon of naturally occurring changes in vaginal colonization over time.

An approach that reduces the number of patients needing screening has been suggested by Minkoff and Mead (1986). They favor culturing all women admitted in preterm labor or with preterm premature amniorrhexis (less than 37 weeks' gestation), and treating with ampicillin those who are either carriers of group B streptococci or those who persist in labor without the available test results.

It has been suggested that a single dose of benzathine penicillin can prevent disease among asymptomatic colonized infants; however, that claim has not been proved, and the approach does not reduce the problem of early-onset disease. Topical care of the umbilical stump can possibly reduce some nosocomial infection in the nursery, as can reemphasis of handwashing as a barrier to contact transmission.

One possible preventative approach may relate to research studies directed at purifying the type-specific group B streptococcal antigens and then measuring maternal antibodies by serologic testing. Risk for newborn disease due to group B streptococci has been correlated with deficiency of specific antibodies in mother–baby pairs. Once a standardized reliable test is generally available for measuring susceptibility to infection, selective vigorous antibiotic treatment can be directed at colonized susceptible individuals. Further research into the immunology of group B streptococcal disease holds promise for development of a vaccine that could be given prior to pregnancy, allowing development of maternal antibodies sufficient to protect the baby by passive transfer during subsequent gestation.

QUESTIONS AND ANSWERS

1. *Should routine antepartum cervical cultures be performed for group B streptococci?*

   This is an option, not a required standard. Although the vaginal colonization rate is high, the neonatal attack rate resulting in severe perinatal infection is relatively low. Thus, colonization of the mother is not often predictive of disease in the baby.

2. *Should an asymptomatic pregnant woman who has been incidentally identified to carry group B streptococci be treated?*

   No. Nevertheless, such information should be recorded for possible intrapartum management and transmitted to the pediatrician at time of delivery. Such information would be particularly helpful if labor were complicated by premature or prolonged amniorrhexis, fever, or premature birth.

SELECTED READINGS

Allardice, J., et al. Perinatal group B streptococcal colonization and infection. *Am. J. Obstet. Gynecol.* 142:617–620, 1982.

Baker, C. Summary of the workshop on perinatal infections due to group B streptococcus. *J. Infect. Dis.* 136:137–152, 1977.

Baker, C., Barrett, F., and Yow, M. The influence of advancing gestation on group B streptococcal colonization in pregnant women. *Am. J. Obstet. Gynecol.* 122:820–823, 1975.

Baker, C., Clark, D., and Barrett, F. Selective broth medium for isolation of group B streptococci. *Appl. Microbiol.* 26:884–885, 1973.

Baker, C., and Kasper, D. Group B streptococcal vaccines. *Rev. Infect. Dis.* 7:458–467, 1985.

Boyer, K., and Gotoff, S. Prevention of early-onset neonatal group B streptococcal disease with selective intrapartum chemoprophylaxis. *N. Engl. J. Med.* 314:1665–1669, 1986.

Minkoff, H., and Mead, P. An obstetric approach to the prevention of early-onset group B β-hemolytic streptococcal sepsis. *Am. J. Obstet. Gynecol.* 54:973–977, 1986.

Yow, M.D., et al. Ampicillin prevents intrapartum transmission of group B streptococcus. *J.A.M.A.* 241:1245–1247, 1979.

14

Urinary Tract Infections

Acute pyelonephritis during pregnancy may cause premature delivery and maternal septicemia. In more recent years, asymptomatic bacteriuria during pregnancy has been recognized as a risk factor for subsequent cystitis or pyelonephritis.

FREQUENCY

Asymptomatic bacteriuria, defined as the confirmed presence of $\geq 10^5$ bacteria per ml of urine occurs during pregnancy, with a prevalence of 2 to 10 percent. The frequency with which such bacteriuria can be detected increases with decreasing socioeconomic class. Black women with sickle hemoglobin have asymptomatic bacteriuria during pregnancy approximately twice as often as black women of the same socioeconomic class who do not have any sickle hemoglobin. Pregnancy itself, diabetes, and parity have not been shown to be related to consistent changes in the incidence of bacteriuria.

Approximately 20 to 30 percent of pregnant women with asymptomatic bacteriuria will develop symptomatic urinary tract infections during pregnancy if the bacteriuria is left untreated. The expected overall rate of symptomatic urinary tract infection in pregnancy is, therefore, less than 3 percent. In the preantibiotic era, patients with symptomatic infection were at high risk for developing potentially fatal sepsis, with premature labor noted as part of a severely morbid clinical situation.

While it has been shown that premature labor can be expected in some pregnant women who have acute pyelonephritis, the pathophysiology of such premature parturition remains unclear. A pregnant woman who has been treated for antepartum pyelonephritis has a recurrence risk of approximately 20 percent for another episode of pyelonephritis. If the mother has been treated successfully with antibiotics, and preterm delivery has been avoided, there is not an increased risk that the fetus will have an adverse outcome.

Claims regarding a proposed increased incidence of prematurity and associated problems in patients who have asymptomatic bacteriuria remain unproved. While it is logical to project an increased risk based on the known sequence of disease progression following asymptomatic bacteriuria, it is difficult to prove the point in clinical studies. The rate of false-positive urine cultures is sufficiently high (1 percent or more), and the overall incidence of prematurity is sufficiently low, that a very large number of pregnant patients with asymptomatic bacteriuria would be required to establish a statistically significant finding.

In addition to prematurity, it is possible that maternal bacteriuria may affect the baby in other ways. It has been suggested that fetal defects of dorsal midline fusion may be found with increased frequency when there has been maternal bacteriuria during early pregnancy; however, the proposed association requires further investigation. The rate of urinary tract infection in newborns is approximately 1 percent at term. A 2- to 10-fold increase in the urinary tract infection rate can be found among premature infants.

Table 14-1. Diagnosis of Urinary Tract Infection

Mother	Child
Clinical	
Asymptomatic bacteriuria Lower tract infection Dysuria Frequency Urgency Low abdominal pain and tenderness Low-grade fever and chills Upper tract infection Lower tract findings can be present Prominent fever and chills Lumbar pain Costovertebral angle tenderness Nausea, vomiting, diarrhea	Asymptomatic bacteriuria Nonspecific signs and symptoms (see Chap. 16, Neonatal Sepsis) Localizing manifestations can include tenderness and swelling in males with infection involving the testicle or epididymis
Laboratory	
Microscopic evidence of significant bacteriuria in fresh urine: Unspun >1–2 WBC/HPF >1–2 bacteria/OPF Spun >10 bacteria/HPF >5 bacteria/OPF Quantitative culture $\geq 10^5$ CFU/ml (single species)	Bag collection specimen Negative culture of $< 10^5$ CFU/ml usually excludes infection Suprapubic aspiration Any growth on culture can be significant, but $> 10^5$ CFU/ml usually found with clinical disease Any bacteria seen by microscopy are significant Examination for leukocytes is not diagnostic

DIAGNOSIS

Mother

Asymptomatic bacteriuria is diagnosed by the presence of a single species of bacteria with a concentration $\geq 10^5$ organisms/ml urine on two consecutive cultures. Pyuria (Table 14-1), an associated finding, is present in approximately one-third of cases. Direct microscopic examination of freshly collected urine for bacteria can be valuable. The finding of >1–2 bacteria/oil power field of unspun urine is strongly correlated with $\geq 10^5$ colony forming units (CFU)/ml upon culturing of the specimen. While various protocols for microscopy can be used, Jenkins and associates (1986) have suggested that oil-immersion microscopy of gram-stained centrifuged urine sediment produces the highest combination of sensitivity and specificity for bacteriuria.

The number of false-positive urine cultures may be as low as 4 percent when there has been optimal collection technique, specimen transportation, and laboratory processing. A clean-catch voided urine specimen is strongly preferred to a catheter specimen in routine circumstances, even if thorough instruction of the patient is required to get a contamination-free specimen. The risk of introducing bacteria into the bladder by catheterization makes catheterization for routine purposes relatively undesirable during pregnancy.

Escherichia coli account for 90 percent of urinary tract infections. *Klebsiella-Enterobacter, Proteus,* and *Enterococcus* predominate among the remainder. A mixed culture usually suggests specimen contamination rather than infection. While quantitative urine culture by plate count technique remains the most reliable laboratory method, a number of alternative methods have been proposed, which an individual practitioner or laboratory may find useful for screening purposes. Such methods are designed to obtain a standardized aliquot of urine for incubation in a variety of special devices that require minimal space and handling. Possibly useful techniques include a filter paper method, a dip slide method, and a pipette method.

A variety of indirect tests for bacteria in urine are available. All can aid in screening patients for subsequent urine culture, but no indirect technique is sufficient to supplant culture quantitation. Tests in use are based on predicted bacterial metabolism, specifically (1) consumption of urine glucose, (2) reduction of nitrate to nitrite, and (3) bacterial dehydrogenase activity. Immunofluorescent staining of urinary sediment may prove useful in predicting patient risk based on the source (kidney versus bladder) of bacteriuria. The technique is based on the observation that bacteria coming from the kidneys are coated with antibody, while bacteria originating in the bladder are not.

Signs and symptoms of maternal pyelonephritis include fever, chills, and pain and tenderness at the costovertebral angle. Cystitis, on the other hand, is characterized by urgency, frequency, dysuria, and suprapubic pain without fever. Fever and the anatomic location of the pain and tenderness are the findings most commonly used to tentatively distinguish cystitis from pyelonephritis. Since symptomatic infections of the bladder and one or both kidneys may coexist, presenting symptoms may vary. In acute pyelonephritis, there may be abdominal pain, nausea, and vomiting in addition to the costovertebral angle pain and tenderness usually expected. Increased uterine activity developing subsequent to or coincident with urinary tract findings may mask the clinical findings of urinary tract infection.

In less severely ill patients, cystitis symptoms may be obscured by the patient's sensations of pelvic pressure and urgency produced by normal pregnancy. As in the nonpregnant patient, symptoms caused by vaginitis and urethritis may be mistaken for dysuria and frequency.

Laboratory tests to confirm symptomatic urinary tract infection include quantitative culture (same criteria as for asymptomatic infection) and microscopic examination of urine for bacteria and leukocytes. Pyuria is a more reliable laboratory finding in the presence of symptomatic infection than when the patient is asymptomatic.

Child

The signs of urinary tract infection in the newborn are nonspecific. Asymptomatic infection may occur more often than symptomatic disease. Clinical manifestations in the first week are those findings consistent with neonatal sepsis. Indeed, it is likely that most neonatal urinary tract infections occur secondary to bacteremia. There may be localized signs of infection in some cases.

When urinary tract infection is suspected, or when sepsis is being evaluated, the optimal method to obtain a specimen for urine culture in current practice is to perform a suprapubic needle aspiration of the bladder. Any growth of a single species of bacteria obtained using this technique is considered significant, excluding obvious contamination at the time of sampling. Microscopic examination of urine for leukocytes or red blood cells has little predictive value in the newborn.

A less invasive technique for collection of urine from newborns involves external washing and application of a plastic collecting bag. The contamination problem with this technique substantially weakens the significance of a positive culture but increases the clinical value of a negative culture for excluding a urinary tract infection.

MANAGEMENT

Mother

Pregnant women with proven asymptomatic bacteriuria should be treated with antibiotics and retreated as often as necessary to maintain a negative urine culture. Acceptable proof of bacteriuria will vary according to clinical circumstances. If there has been a high rate of false-positive cultures, or if an indirect screening test for bacteriuria has been used, the clinician may wish to withhold treatment pending confirmation of the original test result by a quantitative bacterial culture. The consequences of delayed therapy must be weighed against overtreatment based on false-positive results.

Antibiotic therapy for asymptomatic bacteriuria significantly reduces the rate of pyelonephritis in pregnancy. Proper management will prevent 70 to 80 percent of pyelonephritis in pregnant women. This estimate is based on screening all pregnant women for bacteriuria at the time of the first antenatal visit. Such a reduction in morbidity is one of the benefits of beginning obstetric care early in pregnancy.

The choice of antibiotic (Table 14-2) is guided by the result of sensitivity testing, when available. Tetracycline and chloramphenicol are excluded from use during pregnancy. Low cost and proven efficacy against the bacteria that cause the greatest number of infections favor use of a short-acting sulfonamide (e.g., sulfisoxazole) or nitrofurantoin. Both drugs may cause hemolytic anemia in patients with glucose-6-phosphate dehydrogenase deficiency. Additionally, the sulfonamides may contribute to kernicterus in newborns by competing with bilirubin for binding sites; therefore, it is appropriate to avoid prescribing sulfonamides for pregnant women after the 24th week of gestation. Although some have advised that sulfonamides can be given until two weeks prior to term, there is sufficient uncertainty concerning the time of delivery in any gravida that it may be best to avoid sulfonamides once the baby has neared the age of possible viability.

For treating asymptomatic maternal bacteriuria, it has been customary to prescribe 14 days of oral antibiotic therapy. This will clear bacteriuria in 80 percent of patients. A 7 to 10-day course of treatment may be sufficient. Single dose (e.g., amoxicillin 3 g orally) bolus therapy has been shown to be effective in gynecologic cases, and may be shown to be effective and safe for obstetric use provided the patient has adequate follow-up. In any case it is the physician's responsibility to check to be sure that the culture has become negative and that it remains negative.

The 20 percent of patients who do not respond to initial therapy for bacteriuria will need further treatment based on sensitivity testing.

Table 14-2. Management of Urinary Tract Infection

Mother	Child
Treatment*	
Asymptomatic bacteriuria or cystitis First 20 weeks: 14 days of oral antibiotic treatment as guided by sensitivity testing if available, otherwise: *Sulfisoxazole,* 2–4 g initially, then 4–8 g/day in 4–6 divided doses *Nitrofurantoin,* 200–400mg/day in 4 divided doses *Ampicillin,* 2 g/day in 4 divided doses *Cephalexin,* 2g/day in 4 divided doses 2nd 20 weeks: delete sulfisoxazole Acute pyelonephritis Hospitalize to begin parenteral antibiotics, bedrest, and antipyretics Use sensitivity testing to guide antibiotic therapy if available, otherwise: *Ampicillin,* 2 g IV initially, then 1 g q 6 hr *Cephalothin,* 2 g IV initially, then 1 g q 6 hr Switch to oral antibiotics as appropriate when sensitivity test results available and patient afebrile. Continue for 14 days of antibiotic treatment or for the remainder of the pregnancy	Parenteral antibiotics (see Chap. 16, Neonatal Sepsis)
Follow-up	
Check urinalysis for absence of bacteria after 48 hr therapy. Suspect inadequate treatment if bacteria present Repeat urine culture 2 weeks after finishing antibiotics; every 4 6 weeks until delivery; third post-partum day; 6 weeks post partum; and 6 months post partum Treat again if bacteriuria diagnosed Post partum intravenous pyelogram (6–12 weeks) if Acute pyelonephritis during pregnancy Recurrent cystitis Recurrent bacteriuria	Repeat urine culture after treatment completed at 2 weeks; 1, 2, and 3 months; 6 months. Retreat if bacteriuria diagnosed Intravenous pyelogram Soon after initial diagnosis and treatment Vesicourethrogram After infection controlled Specialty consultation for management of anatomic abnormalities

*Do not use chloramphenicol or tetracycline

Fifteen percent of patients will have recurrent bacteriuria after initially successful treatment. Sensitivity testing should guide repeat treatment in these patients. While the majority of these patients can be successfully treated with 14-day courses of antibiotics, a few may require continuous antibiotic treatment for the remainder of pregnancy.

Afebrile patients with cystitis and patients with asymptomatic bacteriuria may be treated as outpatients with oral antibiotics. However, febrile pregnant patients with urinary tract infections should be treated in the hospital. Management should begin with bed rest with lateral positioning to promote drainage of the collecting system of the infected kidney, and intravenous antibiotic and fluid therapy. Antipyretics should be given to keep maternal oral temperature below 39° C (101.5° F). Obstetrical management may include tocolytic agents in order to inhibit premature labor, provided that the clinical diagnosis of urinary tract infection has been well established and it is reasonably certain that intrauterine infection is not present. If the cause of maternal pyrexia and premature labor is unclear, amniocentesis under sonographic guidance is recommended to obtain a specimen for microscopic examination and culture. If the unspun amniotic fluid contains bacteria and leukocytes, the baby should be delivered.

After completion of the initial course of antibiotic therapy for pyelonephritis during pregnancy, a decision must be made either to observe the patient for evidence of recurrent infection or continue antimicrobial therapy. The recurrence rate of pyelonephritis during pregnancy can be significantly reduced by continuing antimicrobial treatment for the remainder of pregnancy (Harris and Gilstrap, 1974); however, the risk of recurring pyelonephritis also may be minimized by monitoring the patient's urine for the return of bacteriuria and then restarting antimicrobial therapy before symptoms develop.

A comparison of short-term and continuous antimicrobial therapy for treatment of asymptomatic bacteriuria has been reported (Whalley and Cunningham, 1977). The cure rate in the continuous treatment group was 88 percent, while in the short-term treatment group 65 percent became abacteriuric for the remainder of pregnancy after one course of therapy, and another 19 percent remained abacteriuric after the second course of therapy. The rates of pyelonephritis during pregnancy were similar in both groups. Thus, both treatment plans seemed equally effective, and the short-term plan seemed preferable for minimizing both risk and expense.

Post-partum follow-up of patients who were treated for a urinary tract infection during pregnancy should include a urine culture on the third post-partum day, and a repeat culture at time of the 4 to 6 week checkup. As part of follow-up assessment for possible renal parenchymal disease, an intravenous pyelogram (IVP) should be performed on all patients who have had an episode of pyelonephritis during pregnancy, recurrent urinary tract infection, or recurrent bacteriuria. The IVP should not be performed until there has been an adequate opportunity for normal pregnancy-related anatomic dilation changes in the urinary collecting system to return to normal (6–12 weeks).

Child

Newborn management should include culture of the blood and spinal fluid in addition to urine culture obtained as part of the workup for possible neonatal sepsis. (See Chap. 16, Neonatal Sepsis.) Systemic antibiotic therapy for the infant suspected of having sepsis is sufficient to cover the possible urinary tract infection. While initial therapy may require high doses of more than one antibiotic when the results of cultures are available, a lower dose of a single agent may be substituted.

An IVP should be considered in the management of a newborn with a proven urinary tract infection, as part of a search for possible structural abnormalities. A vesicourethrogram can be undertaken as an extension of that workup after the infection has been controlled. The yield of anatomic abnormalities demonstrated by such studies will be small, as the majority of neonatal urinary tract infections seems to be secondary to sepsis rather than to ascending infection.

PREVENTION

The great majority of symptomatic urinary tract infections could be prevented if asymptomatic bacteriuria were diagnosed and successfully treated. Ideally, such prevention would be facilitated during pregnancy by performing a series of urine cultures; however, there is not a uniform policy in practice concerning urine cultures for asymptomatic women.

In the minimal surveillance culture programs common in obstetric practice in the United States, quantitative urine cultures are performed only when there is some evidence of unusual risk such as a history of prior urinary tract infections, sickle hemoglobin, or when a routine urinalysis is abnormal. More ambitious programs include an indirect test for bacteriuria as a criterion for obtaining a urine culture. Further clinical management studies are needed in this area.

QUESTIONS AND ANSWERS

1. *What can be done for a pregnant woman with pyelonephritis who goes into premature labor?*

   Continue intravenous antibiotic therapy for pyelonephritis and add best available drug for tocolysis. Regimens in use in the United States include alcohol, magnesium sulfate, ritodrine, or terbutaline.

2. *Prior to pregnancy, postcoital urinary tract infections were successfully suppressed by single-dose postcoital antibiotic treatment. What should be done during pregnancy?*

   If the patient has coitus she should continue the antibiotic treatment. If she was taking a sulfonamide, then ampicillin, cephalexin, or nitrofurantoin would be preferable during the last half of pregnancy. The patient should be evaluated for asymptomatic bacteriuria at least once in each trimester and again on the third day post partum.

SELECTED READINGS

Bergstrom, T., et al. Studies of urinary tract infection in infancy and childhood XII. Eighty consecutive patients with neonatal infection. *J. Pediatr.* 80:858–866, 1972.

Gilstrap, L., Cunningham, F., and Whalley, P. Acute pyelonephritis in pregnancy: An anterospective study. *Obstet. Gynecol.* 57:409–413, 1981.

Gilstrap, L., et al. Renal infection and pregnancy outcome. *Am. J. Obstet. Gynecol.* 141:709–716, 1981.

Harris, R., and Gilstrap, L. Prevention of recurrent pyelonephritis during pregnancy. *Obstet. Gynecol.* 44:637–641, 1974.

Jenkins, R., Fenn, J., and Matsen, J. Review of urine microscopy for bacteriuria. *J.A.M.A.* 255:3397–3403, 1986.

Leveno, K., et al. Bladder versus renal bacteriuria during pregnancy: Recurrence after treatment. *Am. J. Obstet. Gynecol.* 139:403–406, 1981.

Norden, C., and Kass, E. Bacteriuria of pregnancy—A critical appraisal. *Ann. Rev. Med.* 19:431–470, 1968.

Whalley, P., and Cunningham, F. Short-term versus continuous antimicrobial therapy for asymptomatic bacteriuria in pregnancy. *Obstet. Gynecol.* 49:262–265, 1977.

15

Chorioamnionitis

Chorioamnionitis is strictly defined as inflammation of the chorion and amnion demonstrated by leukocytic infiltration of the membranes. In clinical obstetrics the term chorioamnionitis has broader meaning, which includes infection of the uterus, fetus, and amniotic fluid. When untreated, such infection can progress to sepsis that is potentially lethal for mother and baby.

FREQUENCY

Neutrophils and bacteria can be found on histologic examination of the chorion and amnion following 10 to 20 percent of all deliveries. The frequency of histologic chorioamnionitis is inversely proportional to birth weight, and may exceed 50 percent in the membranes of infants weighing less than 2000 g at birth. While the frequency of histologic chorioamnionitis is more than 10 times the overall incidence of clinically manifest chorioamnionitis, in nearly all fatal cases of fetal intrauterine bacterial infection, histologic chorioamnionitis is present.

Premature amniorrhexis, or rupture of the membranes before the onset of labor, is significantly related to histologic chorioamnionitis, clinical chorioamnionitis, and prematurity. Usually, the cause of premature amniorrhexis is not known, although infection of the endocervix, decidua, and adjacent membranes can cause membrane rupture in some cases. Labor usually begins within 24 hours once amniorrhexis has occurred. At term, the expected rate of prompt spontaneous labor following amniorrhexis is approximately 90 percent, while with increasing prematurity, the rate of spontaneous labor within 24 hours falls by approximately one-half. Nonetheless, if labor is not induced, spontaneous labor will have occurred within three days in approximately 70 percent of preterm pregnancies with ruptured membranes. Labor will have begun in more than 90 percent of such pregnancies within two weeks from the onset of amniorrhexis. Thus, when premature amniorrhexis occurs before 34 weeks' gestation, premature birth should be expected.

The incidence of both histologic and clinical chorioamnionitis increases with the duration of amniorrhexis; however, precise measurement of the incidence of clinical chorioamnionitis is difficult because of imprecision in the end point being studied. If fever during labor is used as the end point implying clinical chorioamnionitis, less than 2 percent of an unselected series of patients should have fever during labor. In patients with premature amniorrhexis the overall incidence of fever during labor is approximately 10 percent, rising to 25 percent or more when the duration of amniorrhexis has exceeded 24 hours. This material febrile morbidity is usually inversely related to socioeconomic status. The reason for such an association is not known, but a range of factors, including poor nutrition, decreased amniotic fluid inhibitors of bacterial growth, poor prenatal care, and more preexisting infection, have been suggested as possible partial explanations.

The natural consequence of untreated intrapartum chorioamnionitis is puerperal endometritis. This complication is common if there has been an operative delivery. Although some studies have shown little or no increased fetal risk following premature amnior-

Table 15-1. Diagnosis of Chorioamnionitis

Clinical

A. Maternal fever most common sign
Fetal tachycardia (> 180) usually present with maternal fever
B. May be present:
1. Chills
2. Uterine pain and tenderness
3. Foul vaginal discharge
4. Hypotension
5. Tachycardia

Laboratory

A. Smear of amniotic fluid
Unspun specimen usually shows bacteria and neutrophils
B. Culture of amniotic fluid of uterine cavity
1. Usually mixture of aerobes and anaerobes normally present in endocervix
2. Accepted as pathogens whenever present:
a. *Streptococcus pyogenes* (group A *Streptococcus*)
b. *Neisseria gonorrhoeae*
c. *Staphylococcus aureus*
C. Histology
Chorion and amnion infiltrated with leukocytes
D. Hematology
Increased WBC with > 90 percent polys and bands

rhexis, many studies have shown that the fetal risk for perinatal mortality related to infection increases with the duration of amniorrhexis. Further, it is widely agreed that there is enhanced perinatal mortality subsequent to the onset of symptomatic chorioamnionitis. Perinatal mortality can be expected to range from 2 to 50 percent when the mother has been symptomatic. The mortality increases with decreased gestational age and increased duration of chorioamnionitis.

DIAGNOSIS

The most common clinical manifestation of chorioamnionitis is fever. Other, less consistent, clinical findings include chills, foul vaginal discharge, and uterine pain and tenderness (Table 15-1). Because of the nonspecific nature of the signs and symptoms associated with chorioamnionitis, the diagnosis is usually made by exclusion. A febrile woman in labor is assumed to have chorioamnionitis unless another cause for the fever can be demonstrated.

The diagnostic evaluation of a febrile woman in labor includes a search for evidence of upper respiratory infection, otitis, pneumonia, cystourethritis, pyelonephritis, and phlebitis as the most common extrauterine types of infection. It is important to examine a fresh clean urine specimen for bacilluria and pyuria, as mild pain and tenderness associated with urinary tract infection can be easily confused with or obscured by uterine pain or tenderness during labor. A white blood cell count is usually of minimal value unless the leukocytosis is dramatic ($> 20{,}000/mm^3$) or the predominance of polymorphonuclear leukocytes plus band forms exceed 90 percent of the differential count.

Direct examination of the amniotic fluid can be helpful. The clinical

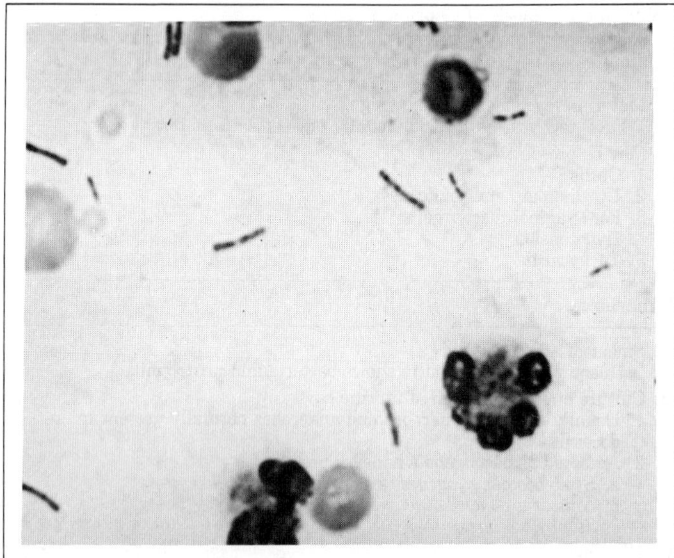

Fig. 15-1. Polymorphonuclear leukocytes and bacteria in amniotic fluid (× 1000).

diagnosis of suspected chorioamnionitis is confirmed when an unspun smear of amniotic fluid from a febrile labor patient shows polymorphonuclear leukocytes and bacteria, provided the specimen was not contaminated by blood or collected from the vagina or endocervix (Fig. 15-1). While specimen collection by amniocentesis is the best method for avoiding vaginal contamination, the usual method for obtaining amniotic fluid for analysis from patients in labor is through an intrauterine open-end polyethylene catheter if one is being used for monitoring intrauterine pressure. A specimen of amniotic fluid obtained for diagnostic microscopic analysis should also be used for culture.

If analysis of amniotic fluid from a febrile patient shows neither neutrophils nor bacteria, the diagnosis of chorioamnionitis can be excluded in the great majority of cases. The exceptions to this rule are infections of the fetus that were transmitted by maternal septicemia and ascending infections through the decidua that reach the placenta without entering the amniotic fluid. Together, these two types of fetoplacental infection should account for less than 5 percent of intrapartum bacterial infections of the uterus.

While the presence of neutrophils and bacteria in the amniotic fluid of a woman in labor may be consistent with the diagnosis of chorioamnionitis, these findings also are common in asymptomatic women. Such patients may have subclinical infection, and they will usually remain asymptomatic if delivered vaginally without trauma. The bacteria recovered from such patients' amniotic fluid represents a sampling of the bacteria found in the endocervix before membrane rupture unless an exogenous organism has been introduced by the obstetrician.

The most common bacteria found are anaerobic streptococci, *Escherichia coli*, aerobic streptococci (not group A), lactobacillus, *Staphylococcus epidermis*, and *Bacteroides* species. It has been suggested (Gibbs et al., 1985) that the bacteria isolated from the amniotic fluid can be categorized as either high- or low-virulence organisms. They report that when high-virulence bacteria were present and a cesarean delivery occurred the rate of endometritis was greater than 90 percent, compared to a puerperal endometritis rate of approximately 46 percent if there was vaginal delivery. Although anaerobic streptococci have been traditionally described as the most frequent anaerobes associated with endometritis, the role of various *Bacteroides* species has been highlighted in studies that used sufficient technical precautions to obtain a high yield of fastidious anaerobes from clinical samples.

Although perinatal infections due to clostridia are reported somewhat less frequently now than in the past, they merit specific comment. Rarely, certain members of the genus *Clostridium* (*C. perfringens, C. septicum, C. novyi*) are recovered from genital flora. Clostridial infections may be associated with prolonged intrauterine demise in the second and third trimesters or criminal septic incomplete abortions. These patients show signs of septicemia frequently with superimposed disseminated coagulopathy, hemolysis, or renal failure. Hemolysis of red blood cells may produce a characteristic "port wine" serum and urine, and there may be hyperkalemia due to cell necrosis. This may be aggravated by renal failure due to shock. X-rays may show evidence of bacterial generation of subcutaneous gas.

Septic pelvic thrombophlebitis is an occasional complication of anaerobic pelvic infections. The diagnosis is usually established by exclusion. Classically, patients with this condition develop and consistently maintain a tachycardia out of proportion to their pyrexia despite broad-spectrum, multiple-drug chemotherapy. Frequently no significant pelvic findings are present except for diffuse uterine and adnexal tenderness without masses. Venous cords may infrequently be palpable at pelvic examination. Occasionally, there is unilateral groin tenderness in the femoral triangle. Contrary to earlier teaching, septic pelvic thrombophlebitis is not exclusively associated with any specific type of anaerobic organism (e.g., anaerobic streptococci). A CAT scan of the pelvis can be a valuable diagnostic tool to show clots in the iliac vessels. The patient's rapid clinical response when heparin therapy is instituted confirms the diagnosis.

There is general agreement that delivery trauma that produces a hematoma or devitalized tissue facilitates the development of maternal infection. For example, cesarean section performed after the amniotic fluid has been contaminated by bacteria and subclinical infection has developed is one of the more common causes of puerperal infection in current obstetric practice.

In a minority of women, the initial manifestations of chorioamnionitis will progress to include hypotension, tachycardia, and oliguria when significant maternal systemic infection has occurred. In such cases there is usually fetal sepsis and there may be microabscesses in the myometrium.

The most common fetal manifestation of chorioamnionitis is tachycardia (fetal heart rate greater than 180); however, this is a nonspecific finding that is secondary to maternal fever regardless of cause and is not diagnostic of disease in the baby. The full-term fetus can usually tolerate 6 to 10 hours of exposure to contaminated amniotic fluid before birth without a major proven increased incidence of infection. The colonization attack ratio may be as high as 50:1, but awaits further clinical research clarification. When clinical infection of the baby does occur, manifestations may include death in utero, congenital pneumonia, newborn sepsis, and meningitis. (See Chaps. 13 and 16, Group B Streptococcal Infections and Neonatal Sepsis.)

The laboratory identification of the bacteria present in specific cases of chorioamnionitis or puerperal endometritis is a time-consuming process that will not provide answers until after the majority of patients have been successfully treated by early empiric broad-spectrum antimicrobial therapy. Nevertheless, clinicians will need culture results to guide the diagnosis and therapy of patients who did not respond to initial measures, particularly when an anaerobic infection is suspected.

If certain practices are observed, reasonably adequate recovery of anaerobes can be accomplished in a clinical setting. Ideally, specimens should be immediately plated on selected blood agar plates maintained in anaerobic jars either at the bedside or following prompt transport to the laboratory. Although these practices may be logistically impossible, such circumstances do not eliminate the likelihood of reasonably good anaerobic recovery of clinically significant organisms. In puerperal endometritis cases, double or triple lumen swab devices have been used effectively to get a sample of the endometrial cavity at the time of a pelvic examination while minimizing contamination from the vagina and adjacent cervix.

Various transport systems, including gassed oxygen-free tubes with swabs or Stuart transport medium with charcoal and added agar may be used to deliver specimens to the laboratory. Such carrying systems should be fresh, and delay in transport time to the laboratory should be minimized. Specimens in transit should be kept out of direct light and not be permitted to dry out because desiccation, especially in association with oxidation, rapidly kills anaerobes. In the absence of liquid pus, perhaps the best transport medium is the tissue itself in which an anaerobic infection is suspected. If liquid pus is present, it should be drawn up in a glass syringe, capped, and promptly transported to the laboratory for processing. It is most important that laboratory personnel be advised that specimens should be specifically processed for anaerobic growth, since the majority of organisms successfully delivered to the bacteriology laboratory can be recovered with meticulous microbiologic technique.

Since most anaerobes grow slowly, especially if they are competing in comparatively small numbers with other organisms for nutrients, it is imperative that the laboratory holds all inoculated culture media for a minimum of 8 days and preferably 10 to 14 days before reporting that there is no growth. This delay underscores the clinical importance of a Gram's stain of material obtained at the time of culturing to guide the initial therapy.

MANAGEMENT

The essence of management of symptomatic chorioamnionitis is delivery of the baby (Table 15-2). Atraumatic vaginal delivery is preferred to cesarean section or difficult midforceps delivery, and it is usually acceptable to wait for several hours for an atraumatic vaginal delivery if there has been satisfactory progress in labor rather than to intervene with an early cesarean section. While some physicians would wait 12 hours for vaginal delivery, 6 to 8 hours seems to be a

Table 15-2. Management of Chorioamnionitis

A. Delivery is essential
   1. Atraumatic vaginal delivery preferred
   2. Allow 6–8 hours of continued labor with antibiotic treatment in presence of
      a. Mild infection
      b. Satisfactory rate of cervical dilation and descent of presenting part
   3. Prompt delivery by cesarean section, if necessary, when there is
      a. Severe infection
      b. Dystocia, or small likelihood of vaginal delivery within 8 hours
      c. Fetal distress

B. Antibiotics
   1. Avoid chloramphenicol, sulfas, and tetracyclines
      Culture blood and uterus or amniotic fluid before starting drug
      Adjust treatment later based on culture results
   2. *Mild Infection.* One drug
      Ampicillin or cephalothin, 1–2 g IV every 4–6 hr until afebrile for 24 hr, then continue with oral antibiotic for completion of 7 days treatment or until afebrile for 48–72 hr. Oral ampicillin, 500 mg every 6 hr. Since cephalothin is not given orally, cephalexin may be used, 500 mg every 6 hr
   3. *Severe Infection.* A single cephalosporin with efficacy against anaerobes, or a combination of two or three drugs. Usual duration of treatment 7 days or until afebrile for 48–72 hr. Drugs may be given orally, if available, as tolerated after patient has become afebrile for 24 hr
      a. Cefoxitin 2 g IV every 6 hr
      b. Clindamycin 1200 to 2700 mg/day IV in divided doses *plus* gentamicin or tobramycin 5 mg/kg/day IM or IV in divided doses
      c. Ampicillin 4–12 g/day IV or penicillin G 10–30 million U/day IV *plus* gentamicin or tobramycin *plus* clindamycin

more acceptable maximum waiting period in current practice. Nonetheless, if the clinical outlook for expeditious labor and vaginal delivery is unfavorable at the time clinical chorioamnionitis has been diagnosed, it is better to proceed with a prompt cesarean section than to wait for further confirmation of dystocia while the infection becomes more severe.

Intravenous antibiotic treatment should be started promptly for a woman with confirmed symptomatic chorioamnionitis. The treatment regimen will vary with the severity of infection. If the patient's fever is lower than 39° C (102.2° F) and she does not have striking associated clinical findings of profound infection, a single antibiotic is usually adequate treatment. One or two grams of ampicillin or a first-generation cephalosporin such as cefazolin can be given intravenously every four to six hours. When the patient seems severely ill, as manifest by a temperature higher than 40° C (104° F) or clinical signs of septic shock, more extensive antibiotic treatment with multiple antibiotics or a cephalosporin with good coverage of anaerobes such as cefoxitin is recommended. Acceptable combinations include an aminoglycoside and clindamycin or a penicillin with an aminoglycoside and clindamycin (Table 15-2).

When cesarean section is needed for delivery of a patient with chorioamnionitis, the transperitoneal approach usually produces satisfactory results. The extraperitoneal approach has been recommended by some. The idea that contaminated amniotic fluid and blood will be excluded from spilling into the peritoneal cavity is tempting, but the extraperitoneal technique is difficult to perform properly and few obstetricians have been trained in its use.

The most severely infected patients may need to be delivered by cesarean hysterectomy in order to prevent death from sepsis. The added risk of cesarean hysterectomy is warranted when myometritis appears to have progressed to multiple abscesses or necrosis with texture suggestive of bacterial gas formation. In such situations, failure to excise these devitalized tissues would leave a substantial source of maternal sepsis that could not be reliably treated with antibiotics alone (See Table 15-2).

PREVENTION

Prevention of epidemic puerperal sepsis by introducing aseptic technique to the delivery process was a major health-care advance in the preantibiotic era. Droplet and contact transmission was interrupted by use of masks, gowns, handwashing, gloves, instrument sterilization, and scrubbing and draping of the patient. Further reduction in the incidence of puerperal sepsis may be due to the widespread use of penicillins in modern medicine. Most epidemics of puerperal sepsis were believed to be due to *Streptococcus pyogenes*, which has remained consistently sensitive to penicillin.

Since most cases of clinical chorioamnionitis in current practice are due to endogenous infection by combinations of bacteria that are otherwise a part of normal endocervical flora, efforts to prevent chorioamnionitis and post-partum endometritis have been directed toward interrupting the progression from colonization to disease. One approach has been to use parenteral broad-spectrum antibiotics for cesarean-section patients. Studies that have examined the use of prophylactic antibiotics for cesarean-section patients have consistently demonstrated approximately 50 percent reduction in postpartum maternal infection-related morbidity (measured as febrile morbidity, fever index, or the incidence of clinically suspect endometritis). Some studies have shown a shorter duration of hospital stay in patients who received prophylaxis. Although this has led to widespread use of antibiotic prophylaxis for cesarean-section patients, the appropriateness of prophylaxis for all cesarean-section patients has remained controversial. It has been said that the benefits sought have been overemphasized, while the risks have not been adequately considered. The morbidity that is reduced by antibiotic prophylaxis is relatively minor in most patients. Life-threatening infectious complications may not be reduced by prophylaxis, while the allergic reactions and infections resistant to the antibiotic given can be major hazards of the prophylaxis regimen.

Prophylactic antibiotics are recommended for those cesarean-section patients whose likelihood of developing symptomatic postpartum infection seems high. Prophylaxis is appropriate for all patients who have had cord prolapse, prolapse of a fetal extremity, or gross contamination of the operative site (e.g., fetal scalp electrode dragged through the operative site). Prophylaxis has also been recommended for afebrile cesarean-section patients whose amniotic fluid smear has shown leukocytes and bacteria. Some call such use of antibiotics early treatment rather than true prophylaxis. The decision to use prophylactic antibiotics can be based on the presence of various risk factors such as labor, amniorrhexis, low socioeconomic status, history of prostitution, drug addiction, or positive gonorrhea culture during pregnancy.

Having decided to give antibiotic prophylaxis, it is recommended that the drug be given intravenously during the cesarean section beginning immediately after birth of the baby. While such a plan gives up the theoretical advantage of having tissue levels of antibiotic before making the decision, the plan seems to work in practice. It allows a culture to be obtained from the uterine cavity if the amniotic fluid was not cultured earlier, and it avoids the confusion of incomplete antibiotic treatment of the baby. A variety of antibiotics have been used for variable treatment periods. Endometrial cavity irrigation with antimicrobial solutions after removal of the placenta has also been shown to be effective in reducing the puerperal endometritis rate.

We have been satisfied with using short-term prophylaxis with either ampicillin or a first- or second-generation cephalosporin. Prophylaxis should be limited to a single-dose regimen or to a multiple-dose regimen that does not exceed 24 hours' duration. If the patient has not been febrile, antibiotics are stopped at that time. Patients who develop symptomatic infections are given full courses of treatment with additional antibiotics as needed.

The decision whether or not to use antibiotic prophylaxis should remain the responsibility of the individual practitioner. Before beginning to use prophylaxis, local statistics should show that significant risk of infection is present. Subsequent ongoing surveillance of infectious morbidity and the bacteriology of wound infections should be maintained.

QUESTIONS AND ANSWERS

1. *If ampicillin, gentamicin, and clindamycin are used in combination for severe chorioamnionitis, why not use all three drugs for mild to moderate infection?*

   One or two antibiotics are sufficient for cure in the great majority of women with chorioamnionitis even though cultures may demonstrate the presence of some species of bacteria resistant to the drugs used. Such good clinical results may be due in large part to the underlying host defense mechanisms of the generally young, healthy, pregnant woman. Use of all three drugs would increase cost as well as risk of allergic reaction and emergence of resistant bacteria.

2. *Can chorioamnionitis be prevented by treating any bacteria recovered from antepartum cervical cultures?*

   Usually not. Exceptions are the gonococcus and, possibly, the Group B *Streptococcus*. (See Chap. 13, Group B Streptococcal Infections.) The large majority of cases of clinical chorioamnionitis is due to bacteria otherwise identified as normal endocervical flora.

SELECTED READINGS

Blanc, W. Amniotic infection syndrome: Pathogenesis, morphology, and significance in circumnatal mortality. *Clin. Obstet. Gynecol.* 2:705–734, 1959.

Cartwright, P., et al. The use of prophylactic antibiotics in obstetrics and gynecology. A review. *Obstet. Gynecol. Surv.* 39:537–554, 1984.

Donowitz, L., and Wenzel, R. Endometritis following cesarean section: A controlled study of the increased duration of hospital stay and direct cost of hospitalization. *Am. J. Obstet. Gynecol.* 137:467–469, 1980.

Gibbs, R., et al. Asymptomatic parturient women with high-virulence bacteria in the amniotic fluid. *Am. J. Obstet. Gynecol.* 152:650–654, 1985.

Gunn, G., Mishell, D., and Morton, D. Premature rupture of the fetal membranes: A review. *Am. J. Obstet. Gynecol.* 106:469–483, 1970.

Hawrylyshyn, P., Bernstein, P., and Papsin, F. Short-term antibiotic prophylaxis in high-risk patients following cesarean section. *Am. J. Obstet. Gynecol.* 145:285–289, 1983.

Larsen, J., et al. Significance of neutrophils and bacteria in the amniotic fluid of patients in labor. *Obstet. Gynecol.* 47:143–147, 1976.

Swartz, W., and Grolle, K. The use of prophylactic antibiotics in cesarean section: A review of the literature. *J. Reprod. Med.* 26:595–609, 1981.

16

Neonatal Sepsis

Neonatal sepsis is a daily concern in any newborn service. While specific causes for sepsis are a recurrent theme in this book, this chapter reviews the general approach to management of the newborn in whom sepsis is suspected in the first four weeks of life.

FREQUENCY

The overall incidence of neonatal sepsis is less than 1 percent of live births; however, the incidence is dramatically skewed by a number of risk factors. The most significant risk factors include intrapartum maternal sepsis or amniotic fluid infection, premature or prolonged amniorrhexis, prematurity, difficult resuscitation, catheterization of umbilical artery or vein, endotracheal intubation, and congenital anomalies. When one or more of these risk factors is present, the incidence of sepsis increases to 30 percent or more especially in very small babies. When sepsis has been definitely proved, the case fatality rate is reported to be approximately 20 to 50 percent. Residual morbidity among survivors depends on the organ systems involved. Pneumonia, urinary tract infection, or meningitis occurs in one-third of septic newborns. Approximately 50 percent of those who survive meningitis may have neurologic impairment.

In contrast to this bleak picture, term neonates who were born without trauma can be exposed to a variety of potentially pathogenic bacteria in the amniotic fluid during labor and yet have a sepsis rate that does not exceed 3 percent. Such babies have some ability to resist both surface and blood bacterial contamination. Studies of cord blood cultures have shown that while the rate of cord blood bacteremia may be 14 to 25 percent, the colonization/disease ratio is only 50:1.

Almost any species of bacteria can cause neonatal sepsis; however, in current practice *Escherichia coli* and group B streptococci account for the great majority of septicemias. Other streptococci, *Staphylococcus aureus, Pseudomonas, Klebsiella, Enterobacter, Proteus, Salmonella* and *Listeria monocytogenes* can cause sepsis in the minority of nonepidemic cases. *Staphylococcus epidermidis* is now recognized as a significant pathogen for neonates, accounting for at least 10 percent of sepsis cases in neonatal intensive care units. Anaerobes are thought to be a rare cause of newborn sepsis, but the reported frequency of sepsis due to anaerobes may be falsely low due to insufficient efforts to culture the organisms.

DIAGNOSIS

Common clinical manifestations of sepsis in the newborn are nonspecific and include minimal changes in alertness and receptivity to feeding that may result in the nurses' warning, "The baby does not seem quite right." (See Table 16-1.) More obvious findings include abdominal distention, gastric residual in gavage-fed babies, vomiting, diarrhea, pallor or icterus, lethargy or irritability, tachypnea, respiratory distress, tachycardia, hypotension, and hepatosplenomegaly. Fever may be present in about one-half of septic older newborns, while hypothermia is more common among septic premature infants. Additional findings consistent with concomitant encephalitis or meningitis are apnea, bulging fontanelle, and seizures.

Table 16-1. Diagnosis of Neonatal Sepsis

Clinical manifestations (can be quite variable)

Decreased alertness or irritability
Decreased receptivity to feeding
- Abdominal distention
- Gastric residual before feeding in gavage-fed babies
- Vomiting
- Diarrhea
- Hepatosplenomegaly
- Weak suck
- Gallbladder distention

Pallor, icterus, or petechiae
Tachypnea or respiratory distress
Tachycardia or hypotension
Hypothermia or fever
With concomitant encephalitis or meningitis
- Apnea
- Bulging fontanelle
- Seizures

Laboratory findings (nonspecific)

White blood cell count <5000 cells/mm^3 or $>25{,}000$ cells/mm^3
Immature to total (I:T) neutrophil ratio ≥ 0.2
Bacteria and leukocytes on smear of gastric aspirate taken just after birth
Changes in acute-phase reactant concentrations
- Increase: Erythrocyte sedimentation rate, C-reactive protein, haptoglobin, orosomucoid
- Decrease: Prealbumin, transferrin

Hyperbilirubinemia (direct)
Disseminated intravascular coagulation (prolonged prothrombin and partial thromboplastin times, decreased platelet counts)
Hypoglycemia
Hyponatremia
Hypocalcemia
Detection of bacterial antigens in cerebrospinal fluid, blood, or urine (by counterimmunoelectrophoresis, latex particle agglutination, or coagglutination methods)

The specific laboratory diagnosis of sepsis is made by a positive blood culture from a symptomatic newborn. Ideally, two positive blood cultures would have been obtained; however, a single blood culture is sufficient when symptoms are severe. Bacteria isolated from septicemia cases include the wide spectrum of gram-positive and gram-negative organisms present in the maternal birth canal as well as organisms that are more often acquired by nosocomial transmission after birth. Nonspecific laboratory tests that can support the diagnosis of sepsis include a white blood cell count fewer than 5000 cells/mm^3 or more than 25,000 cells/mm^3, a differential count that has more than 90 percent cells in the neutrophil series, an increased band count, increased erythrocyte sedimentation rate, hyperbilirubinemia (direct), hypoglycemia, or hyponatremia. Antenatal exposure to bacteria may be demonstrated by stained smear and culture of the amniotic fluid or gastric aspirate.

Analysis of fluid obtained by bladder puncture or by spinal tap may give evidence of specific system infection. Bacilluria seen on a specimen obtained by suprapubic tap is strong evidence of urinary tract infection. Increased spinal fluid protein, spinal fluid leukocytosis, and hypoglycorrhachia are consistent with meningitis. In addition, spinal fluid may be tested for endotoxin by the limulus assay. Immunoelectrophoretic techniques for analysis of the spinal fluid also can give an early warning that bacterial antigens are present.

MANAGEMENT

When neonatal sepsis is suspected, prompt treatment is required to minimize morbidity and potential mortality. Even when clinical manifestations of possible sepsis are minimal, it is desirable to obtain cultures from blood, urine, and spinal fluid, as well as from any discharge, site of gross inflammation, or diarrheal stool. Microscopic examination of stained smears should be included. Vigorous early evaluation of a minimally ill newborn is preferred to delay of the complete workup while awaiting more striking symptoms. While cultures are being obtained, a chest x-ray should be ordered, and an intravenous infusion should be started.

Antibiotic treatment should be started as soon as possible after the specimens for culture and microscopic examination have been obtained. The usual strategy is to begin a combination of ampicillin and an aminoglycoside to cover streptococci, *Listeria*, and enteric gram-negative rods (Table 16-2). Choice of antibiotics will be strongly influenced by local epidemiologic surveillance data as well as clinical considerations such as the age of the newborn at the time the sepsis is suspected. In older newborns, ticarcillin and gentamicin may be the preferred regimen for initial therapy to cover the expected higher incidence of infection due to *Staphylococcus aureus* or resistant gram-negative rods. If bacteria resistant to the usual antibiotic combination have been commonly isolated from patients in a particular nursery, then initial therapy should be adjusted accordingly. It is recommended that such modification of antibiotic selection be made on a hospital-by-hospital basis as indicated from antibiograms compiled from each newborn service.

The recommended initial antibiotic combination of ampicillin and an aminoglycoside does not cover *Pseudomonas, S. aureus,* or *Bacteroides fragilis* well. If aerobic cultures are negative and clinical manifestations of infection continue after 48 hours, ticarcillin or methicillin may be added to the treatment plan, depending on clinical suspicion or available laboratory evidence indicating the most likely resistant organism. If *Pseudomonas* is the etiologic agent, antimicrobial therapy should consist of ticarcillin and an aminoglycoside. *Staphylococcus epidermidis* sepsis is best treated with vancomycin. Multiply resistant gram-negative enteric bacteria may be treated with third-generation cephalosporins such as cefotaxime. Serum concentrations of the aminoglycosides and vancomycin should be carefully monitored since the margin between therapeutic and toxic levels is narrow.

Supportive measures are important in the management of neonatal sepsis, especially the more severe cases. Careful attention to fluid and electrolyte balance, mechanical support of ventilation whenever necessary, and the use of fresh frozen plasma and granulocyte transfu-

Table 16-2. Antibiotic Treatment of Sepsis During the First Week of Life*

Initial treatment when organism unknown and maternal flora suspected

Ampicillin, IV or IM, 25 mg/kg dose q 8 or 12 hr[a]

plus

Kanamycin,[b] IV over 20 min, or IM:

Birthweight < 2000 g	Birthweight > 2000 g
7.5 mg/kg q 12 hr	10.0 mg/kg q 12 hr

or

Gentamicin, IV over 20 min, or IM, 2.5 mg/kg q 12 hr

Pseudomonas or *Bacteroides* suspected

Gentamicin as above

plus

Ticarcillin IV or IM 75 mg/kg q 8 or q 12 hr

Staphylococcus aureus suspected

Methicillin IV

Birthweight < 2000 g	Birthweight > 2000 g
25 mg/kg q 12 hr	25 mg/kg q 8 hr

Coliform shown to be resistant to kanamycin and gentamicin

Tobramycin, IV 4–6 mg/kg/day in divided doses

or

Amikacin, IV, 15 mg/kg/day in divided doses

Staphylococcus epidermidis or methicillin-resistant *Staphylococcus aureus*

Vancomycin 10 mg/kg q 12 hr

*For dosage information beyond the first week of life and for dosage reduction when there is renal failure, see McCracken, G., Jr., and Nelson, J. *Antimicrobial Therapy for Newborns*, 2d ed. New York: Grune and Stratton, 1983.

[a] Double the dose if meningitis is present.

[b] Use gentamicin rather than kanamycin in nurseries where kanamycin-resistant *E. coli* is common.

sions in selected neonates can be very helpful. Removal of foreign bodies that may be sites of colonization may be necessary.

When all cultures have been negative from a reliable laboratory, and the baby seems well, antibiotics may be discontinued if the initial clinical manifestations of possible sepsis were mild or in doubt. If the patient's initial clinical manifestations of infection were severe, then antibiotics should be continued to complete a seven-day course, despite negative cultures. When a positive culture result has been obtained, then one of the antibiotics initially used may be stopped as indicated by sensitivity testing, particularly when the initial clinical manifestations of sepsis were minimal. If there is some doubt regarding the safety of stopping one part of a combination antibiotic regimen, then it it usually better to continue both drugs for a full course of therapy.

PREVENTION

Many of the risk factors related to the likelihood of developing neonatal sepsis are influenced by obstetrical management. It is the obstetrician's responsibility to diagnose and treat antepartum maternal infections, such as pyelonephritis and pneumonia, which have been associated with premature labor. While premature amniorrhexis usually cannot be prevented, early diagnosis will permit a management plan that might attempt to minimize fetal jeopardy. The obstetrical team has a further responsibility to make every reasonable effort to avoid introducing infection to the mother and baby during labor and delivery. Handwashing and sterilized equipment remain major controls against introduction of exogenous infection even in those births for which there has been minimal or no scrubbing and draping of the mother.

Prevention of exogenous infection in the nursery is strengthened by a systematic approach to cleanliness in infant care. Handwashing between patient contacts is an infection-control essential that needs frequent reinforcement by responsible staff members. A cohort system of nursing care and nursery space can have a substantial influence on reducing the epidemic spread of agents such as *S. aureus*. In such a system, the cohort of term babies born on a given day is cared for by one team of nurses and housed in one nursery area until the group of mothers and babies is discharged. When epidemic staphylococcal disease recurs despite these measures, deliberate colonization of newborns with a *Staphylococcus* strain of low virulence has been successful in preventing disease caused by the more virulent organisms (Light et al., 1967).

Water-borne contamination is a well-known source of *Pseudomonas* infection. Possible water-related sources of contamination include skins, soap dispensers, urinalysis equipment, and vaporizers. Intensified surveillance and cleansing of such items usually will substantially reduce the rate of *Pseudomonas* infection.

QUESTIONS AND ANSWERS

1. *Should antibiotics be given prophylactically to newborns who are at high risk for developing sepsis?*

   No. Prophylactic antibiotics have not been shown to change the incidence of sepsis, and prophylaxis makes subsequent diagnosis and treatment of infection more difficult.

2. *Since most sepsis workups do not make a vigorous attempt to culture anaerobes, should routine antibiotic treatment be changed?*

   No. Current therapy is reasonably successful. To change therapy without further study would seem to be unwise.

3. *When should* Staphylococcus epidermis *blood isolates be considered significant rather than mere contaminates?*

   Staphylococcus epidermis sepsis is usually encountered in older neonates, typically those with such risk factors as prematurity, central venous catheters, invasive procedures, and others. If the organism is isolated from both aerobic and anaerobic culture bottles, or if it grows in 72 hours or less, or it is isolated from a second site (e.g., cerebrospinal fluid), then *Staphylococcus epidermis* should be considered pathogenic in the neonate with signs or symptoms of sepsis. Vancomycin is the treatment of choice.

SELECTED READINGS

Berman, N., et al. Cerebrospinal fluid endotoxin concentrations in gram-negative bacterial meningitis. *J. Pediatr.* 88:553–556, 1976.

Chow, A., et al. The significance of anaerobes in neonatal bacteremia: Analysis of 23 cases and review of the literature. *Pediatrics* 54:736–745, 1974.

Light, I., et al. Use of bacterial interference to control a staphylococcal nursery outbreak: Deliberate colonization of all infants with the 502A strain of *Staphylococcus aureus. Am. J. Dis. Child* 113:291, 1967.

McCracken, G., Jr., and Freij, B. Perinatal bacterial diseases. In R. Feigin and J. Cherry (Eds.), *Textbook of Pediatric Infectious Diseases*, 2d ed pp. 940–966. Philadelphia: W.B. Saunders, 1987.

McCracken, G., Jr., and Nelson, J. *Antimicrobial Therapy for Newborns*, 2d ed. New York: Grune and Stratton, 1983.

Siegel, J. Neonatal Sepsis. *Semin. Perinatol.* 9:20–28, 1985.

17 Tuberculosis

Hippocrates first speculated about the interaction between tuberculosis and pregnancy, reputedly ascribing a beneficial effect of motherhood upon "phthisis." Koch isolated the bacillus in 1882. In the late 19th and early 20th centuries, tuberculosis was a common disease and worldwide in distribution. Today, tuberculosis continues to be endemic in southeast Asia and Central and South America. Urban areas, especially those populated by the socioeconomically disadvantaged and immigrants from countries where tuberculosis is endemic, have comparatively high prevalences of active infection. Perhaps for these reasons, Washington, D.C. has the highest case rate for its population of any state or jurisdiction in the continental United States. Congenital tuberculosis, exclusive of neonatal infection from maternal exposure, has been and continues to be a comparatively infrequent clinical event. Nevertheless, failure to diagnose and initiate appropriate therapy for this condition invariably results in significant morbidity and potential mortality for affected infants.

FREQUENCY

Approximately 30,000 new cases of tuberculosis are reported in the United States annually. Estimates show that 1 to 2 percent of pregnant women exhibit tuberculin skin test reactivity. In selected low socioeconomic urban areas, the prevalence of skin test reactivity may be substantially higher, approaching 5 percent. Less than 10 percent of the women in this subpopulation, however, are first diagnosed with active lesions during the index pregnancy. Since approximately half of these women are asymptomatic, estimates of the incidence of active tuberculosis in pregnancy are heavily dependent on the screening techniques employed.

Congenital tuberculosis, requiring carefully documented exclusion of postnatal infection, is uncommon. No correlation exists between the extent of maternal disease and the likelihood that a baby will develop congenital infection. Most congenital tuberculosis results from hematogenous spread of infection from the placenta to the fetus by way of the umbilical vein. Acquisition of infection by aspiration of infected material is a less likely etiology. Nevertheless, the fetus may aspirate infected amniotic fluid in utero, or infected material may be aspirated at the time of birth. Mothers with miliary tuberculosis can bear totally unaffected offspring or systemically septic infants with congenital infection. Alternatively, a single tuberculoma of the endometrium can contaminate amniotic fluid aspirated by the fetus, causing fulminant tuberculous pneumonia and death.

DIAGNOSIS

Mother

Contrary to previous opinion, most women with tuberculosis in pregnancy develop symptoms (Table 17-1). A recent survey demonstrated that only 19 percent of such patients were asymptomatic. Cough (74%), weight loss (41%), fever (30%), malaise and fatigue (30%), and hemoptysis (19%) are frequently presenting signs and symptoms. Fatigue and dyspnea from pulmonary tuberculosis may be difficult to

Table 17.1. Diagnosis of Tuberculosis

Mother	Child
Clinical	
Many are symptomatic Cough Weight loss Fever Malaise Fatigue Hemoptysis	Symptoms are variable Respiratory distress with pneumonitis (usually fulminant) Failure to thrive with hepatosplenomegaly
Laboratory	
Changing pulmonary lesions on serial chest x-rays within six months Recent conversion of PPD Biopsy consistent with diagnosis of tuberculosis with or without isolation of organisms	Positive chest x-rays Altered liver function tests Altered findings in CSF (rare) Positive PPD (after 2–3 months) Isolation of mycobacteria by culture (aspirate) Tissue biopsy compatible with the diagnosis

distinguish from that of pregnancy itself. Physical findings, including pleural effusions, rales, retinopathy, hepatosplenomegaly, and skin lesions are suggestive of the diagnosis but are uncommon. A history of recent tuberculosis exposure should prompt further investigation even among asymptomatic patients. Alternatively, those with symptoms suggestive of tuberculosis from high-risk areas (Southeast Asia, Mexico, Central and South America) should be considered potentially infected, and appropriate diagnostic evaluation must be initiated without delay.

In asymptomatic patients, chest x-rays, especially if earlier comparison films are available, can be extremely helpful. Pulmonary anatomic alterations in pregnancy must be considered in such interpretations. Concerns about fetal risks from irradiation must not deter the physician from obtaining properly shielded views of the chest in any trimester if active clinical disease is suspected. In most series, nearly two-thirds of all patients with pulmonary tuberculosis during pregnancy have evidence of cavitation by x-ray. Ninety percent of such patients demonstrate upper lobe involvement. Tuberculosis skin testing is unaffected by pregnancy but will not identify patients with very early disease or anergy.

Definitive diagnosis requires isolation of mycobacteria from clinical specimens. Since these organisms exhibit notoriously slow growth, the importance of a rapid presumptive diagnosis by direct smear for acid-fast organisms cannot be overemphasized. Most positive smears will show subsequent growth, and therapy should not await cultural verification. In addition to sputa, gastric aspirates and endotracheal washings can be cultured. Depending on the clinical presentation and differential diagnosis, bronchoscopy, mediastinoscopy, scalene node biopsy, liver or pleural biopsy, or bone marrow aspiration may be appropriate. In the event that *Mycobacterium tuberculosis* is successfully isolated from cultures, sensitivities should also be obtained since drug-resistant mycobacteria are being encountered with increasing frequency among current clinical isolates. In one series examining tuberculosis isolates during pregnancy, nearly two-thirds of all infections were caused by "drug-resistant" organisms. In addition to the obvious implications for therapy, identification of such strains is also of prognostic importance. Pregnant women infected with drug-resistant tuberculosis have more extensive roentgenographic abnormalities, longer sputum conversion times, and a higher frequency of pulmonary complications and death compared to those infected with drug-sensitive mycobacteria.

Child

Most children with congenital tuberculosis have no specific symptoms at birth. Occasionally, however, delivery of a premature infant with atypical neonatal sepsis will prompt the consideration of the diagnosis in suggestive clinical settings. Infants who aspirate infected material often develop symptoms within a few days to months following delivery. Without therapy, respiratory distress from severe pneumonia rapidly leads to clinical deterioration and death. Those with nonpulmonic disease may fail to thrive and develop diffuse reticuloendothelial enlargement. In either case, the Mantoux skin test is usually nonreactive until the second or third month of neonatal life. Thus, skin testing is of limited value in establishing the diagnosis of congenital tuberculosis. Absence of skin test reactivity should never be considered to exclude this condition.

Organisms can be isolated from gastric washings of infants, but in many instances the diagnosis is only suggested once the disease is found in the mother. Histologic evidence of placental involvement provides corroborative evidence *only* since both false-positive and false-negative associations are found with congenitally affected offspring. Clinically symptomatic tuberculosis in a mother should be viewed as an indication to carefully and critically evaluate her baby for the presence of congenital infection. Failure to diagnose congenital tuberculosis, resulting in failure to initiate chemotherapy, may result in grave consequences for infected infants.

PROGNOSIS IF UNTREATED

Pregnancy probably does not exert any significant effect on the outcome of maternal tuberculosis. The course of active tuberculosis and the incidence of reactivation is essentially the same in pregnant and nonpregnant patients. Tuberculosis does not increase the incidence of spontaneous abortion or congenital malformation.

Although death from tuberculosis is rare in nondebilitated adults, maternal deaths have occurred in neglected, untreated cases. Fortunately, such instances are rare because progression of the disease usually causes symptoms prompting diagnosis and treatment. The prognosis in undiagnosed neonates is considerably worse. Although spontaneous remissions occasionally occur, untreated congenital tuberculosis usually results in death within weeks to months following the onset of disseminated infection. Thus, for both mother and infant alike, case finding linked to evaluation of those with documented exposure is essential to successful identification of individuals who are infected and the initiation of appropriate therapy.

Table 17-2. Treatment and Follow-up of Tuberculosis

Mother			Child	
Recent PPD conversion but asymptomatic	Active tuberculosis noncavitary 1 lung field	Active tuberculosis extens.	Active tuberculosis	Uninfected but at risk for infection
Treatment				
INH[a] 300 mg PO daily for 6–12 months	INH[a] plus PO daily plus ethambutol 25 mg/kg/day orally for 1 month followed by 10–15 mg/kg/day. Treat for 18 months	INH[a] plus ethambutol plus rifampin 600 mg PO qd for 9 months or for 6 months following sputum conversion, whichever is longer	INH 20 mg/kg/day for one yr. May add ethambutol or rifampin in selected cases	INH prophylaxis or BCG[b] plus careful clinic follow-up
Follow-up				
Quarterly sputum cultures and chest x-rays for all patients with recent skin conversion or active tuberculosis. Skin test and quarterly chest x-rays for uninfected infants at risk for infection from mother				

[a]Supplement with pyridoxine 50 mg PO qd
[b]In high-risk infants of mothers who are noncompliant with therapy

MANAGEMENT

Pregnant and nonpregnant patients alike have a favorable prognosis when given chemotherapy for active tuberculosis. Critical to the successful management of active disease is continuous, prolonged chemotherapy. Because of the emergence of mycobacterial strains resistant to various drugs, combination chemotherapy directed by specific sensitivity testing of isolates is necessary (Table 17-2). Two or more antituberculosis drugs to which the clinical isolate is sensitive should be administered simultaneously to reduce the likelihood of the emergence of drug-resistant organisms.

Patients with recently reactive skin tests should receive isoniazid (INH), 300 mg orally each day, for 6 to 12 months. Pyridoxine, 50 mg orally each day, should be given simultaneously to prevent maternal and fetal neurotoxicity. Pregnant women with noncavitary tuberculosis in one lung field should receive a combination of isoniazid and ethambutol for 18 months. The initial dosage of oral ethambutol is 25 mg/kg/day for the first month of therapy. The dosage of drug may then be reduced to 10 to 15 mg/kg/day. Women with extensive tuberculous disease or those with resistant mycobacterial infections should receive therapy with isoniazid, ethambutol, and rifampin (600 mg a day orally). Therapy should be continued for nine months or for six months after sputum conversion (whichever is longer).

All currently used antituberculous drugs traverse the fetoplacental barrier and are excreted in breast milk. No teratogenic consequences of perinatal isoniazid therapy have been reported. Ethambutol has been associated with cleft palate and central nervous system abnormalities in animals; however, these associations have never been demonstrated in humans. Similarly, rifampin has been associated with spina bifida and cleft palate in rodents when administered at 15 times the normal therapeutic dose. Again, no such association between congenital malformation and drug exposure has been demonstrated during human pregnancies. Streptomycin has been associated with fetal ototoxicity. The extent of damage has ranged from high frequency tone loss to severe deafness. Currently, streptomycin therapy during pregnancy is reserved for rare situations in which the organism responsible for infection is resistant to alternative agents and treatment with streptomycin is essential for successful eradication of infection. In general, following two weeks of adequate chemotherapy, individuals should be considered to be noninfective. Exceptions to this statement apply in cases where extensive cavitary disease is present or when drug-resistant organisms are responsible for infection. Under such circumstances, resolution of infectivity may take as long as six months.

Tuberculosis is spread by aerosolized droplet contamination; therefore, inadequately treated patients in labor who have active tuberculosis should wear masks unless their sputum has been demonstrated by culture to be free of infectious organisms. Whenever there is any question of infectiousness, labor should be conducted in a separate labor room. Local or regional anesthesia to avoid further pulmonary complications is preferable to general.

Breast feeding is not absolutely contraindicated in mothers on chemotherapy. No reports of adverse effects on nursing babies have been made to date. Nevertheless, consideration of the risks and benefits of breast feeding by mothers on therapy should prompt individualized management. Mothers with active disease should not come into contact with their babies if maternal treatment has been given for less than three weeks.

Infants born to mothers with active tuberculosis should be isolated and evaluated to rule out active disease. Chemotherapy, if indicated, should be administered promptly. Even in infants free of disease, chemoprophylaxis with INH should be considered because the baby may be at risk for infection if its mother is inadequately treated. According to estimates, newborns who do not receive antimycotic prophylaxis during the first year of life have a 50 percent risk of contracting acute tuberculosis. In general, offspring of mothers with tuberculosis in pregnancy should receive careful surveillance with skin tests, chest x-rays, and appropriate cultures during the first year of life. Bacillus Calmette Guérin (BCG) vaccination should be given to infants of mothers whose tuberculosis is poorly controlled or who are noncompliant with chemotherapy.

PREVENTION

Early diagnosis is essential in preventing morbidity and mortality from tuberculosis. Actively infected pregnant women and congenitally infected infants will respond favorably in direct proportion to the speed with which correct therapy is instituted. At present no uniformly satisfactory screening procedure is available to detect tuberculosis during pregnancy. Skin testing circumvents the potential fetal hazard of routine chest x-rays. Nevertheless, it is precisely those transient, indigent patients at highest risk who are least likely to return in 48 to 72 hours to have a skin test read. Until alternative approaches are available, a correctly administered skin test must be the minimal requirement in high-risk populations. Patients with a history of exposure or symptoms require both skin testing and roentgenography with shielding.

Once the diagnosis is made, it is crucial that the patient begin adequate chemotherapy without delay. Consultation with a specialist in infectious disease is appropriate in choosing specific drugs, but it is the obstetrician who must assume primary responsibility for patient continuation of chemotherapy and the adequacy of follow-up during pregnancy. Aside from the diagnosis, no other single step is more important in the successful management of tuberculosis in pregnancy.

Intrapartum management of patients under therapy should be planned with the anesthesia staff and nursing personnel in advance, utilizing mask precautions and regional anesthetic techniques as appropriate. Similarly, the pediatric staff must be apprised whenever the diagnosis of tuberculosis is being considered.

Newborns at risk for congenital tuberculosis require isolation and careful follow-up for evidence of infection. Evidence of infection may be delayed in neonates, and maternal illness post partum may warrant prophylactic therapy for the child. Perhaps the most difficult pediatric decision revolves around the administration of BCG, but this is not an acceptable substitute for ongoing case follow-up. Prior to returning home, all family contacts of the mother and child should be surveyed for susceptibility to tuberculosis and treated as appropriate.

Most health advisory agencies have conceded that ultimate control of tuberculosis will only be possible in the distant future. Continued case finding, contact tracing, screening of high-risk patients, and containing and aggressively treating those who are infected are essential steps for successfully eradicating this disease.

QUESTIONS AND ANSWERS

1. *How is a screening skin test for tuberculosis done?*

   Give 5 TU (0.1 ml) of intermediate PPD intradermally and measure the amount of induration that develops after 48 and 72 hours. Ten millimeters or more is considered positive; however, five or more is strongly suggestive in a context of symptoms or known exposure. When 5 TU is used for skin testing, false-negatives will occur. Some false-negative tests will occur in anergic patients with tuberculosis; thus, a negative tuberculosis skin test gains more credence when concurrently performed with a positive control for immunocompromise (for example, mumps, streptokinase-streptodornase, or monilia). The tuberculin (Mantoux) test depends on cell-mediated (delayed) hypersensitivity and may not become positive for up to three months after primary infection. This second important source of false-negatives, women with early disease who have not yet converted their skin test, requires periodic skin test challenge with tuberculin for 12 weeks following the last exposure to rule out active disease. A 100- or 250-TU skin test will rule out tuberculosis in nonanergic individuals once skin test reactivity has developed following primary infection. The risk of extreme skin reactivity with sloughage should be weighed whenever amounts of tuberculin larger than the customary 5-TU screening doses are employed.

2. *Are antituberculosis agents a contraindication to breast feeding?*

   No. However, small amounts of such drugs are secreted in breast milk. Breast feeding was previously thought to aggravate tuberculosis following parturition; however, this has not been substantiated. Breast feeding is contraindicated in instances where mothers are on inadequate chemotherapy, however, as is all mother-child contact until proper treatment can be instituted.

3. *My pregnant patient on INH for recent conversion of her PPD develops unexplained anorexia, nausea, and dark urine. What should I do?*

   These findings (or others such as jaundice, rash, or liver tenderness) should alert the clinician to the possibility of INH-induced hepatitis. Although this is uncommon in patients under the age of 35, suggestive clinical findings require discontinuation of the drug and assessment of liver function with appropriate medical consultation and decisions regarding alternate therapy.

SELECTED READINGS

Cooper, A., Heneghan, W., and Matthew, J. Tuberculosis in a mother and her infant. *Pediatr. Infect. Dis.* 4:181–183, 1985.

Good, J., et al. Tuberculosis in association with pregnancy. *Am. J. Obstet. Gynecol.* 140:492–498, 1981.

Kaplan, C., Benirschke, K., and Tarzy, B. Placental tuberculosis in early and late pregnancy. *Am. J. Obstet. Gynecol.* 137:858–860, 1980.

Kearns, T., and Russo, P. The control and eradication of tuberculosis. *N. Engl. J. Med.* 303:812–814, 1980.

Myers, J., et al. Tuberculosis in pregnancy with fatal congenital infection. *Pediatrics* 67:89–94, 1981.

Nemir, R., and O'Hare, D. Congenital tuberculosis: Review and diagnostic guidelines. *Am. J. Dis. Child.* 139:284–287, 1985.

Niles, R. Puerperal tuberculosis with death of infant. *Am. J. Obstet. Gynecol.* 144:131–132, 1982.

Snider, D., et al. Treatment of tuberculosis during pregnancy. *Am. Rev. Resp. Dis.* 122:65–79, 1980.

18

Listeriosis

Listeria monocytogenes is a motile, gram-positive coccobacillus that causes meningoencephalitis and perinatal infection in ruminants and humans alike. This organism, the causative agent of the neonatal syndrome referred to as *granulomatosis infantiseptica,* was first noted as an epizootic among veldt rodents along the Tiber River in the 1920s. In 1933, Gill described a meningoencephalitis in sheep called *circling disease* caused by *L. monocytogenes*. In the same year, Burn first postulated that listeriosis was a potential perinatal disease after isolating the organism from an infant. In 1951, Reiss and colleagues described the clinical syndrome that has become known as granulomatosis infantiseptica.

FREQUENCY

Listerial meningitis accounts for 1 to 2 percent of all such infections in adults. Listerial infections are rare causes of adult sepsis, endocarditis, and peritonitis. Most adult infections occur among immunosuppressed individuals. Nearly half of all listeriosis in humans occurs in newborns. "Early" neonatal infection, characterized by congenital sepsis, constitutes the majority of such infections. "Late" neonatal infections, characterized by neonatal meningitis, contribute an additional 20 percent of all cases of disease among newborns.

Several recent reports of epidemic listeriosis have contributed to our understanding of the epidemiology of this disease. Although more than 50 different animal species harbor infection (and this agent has caused abortion or meningitis in the majority of these), dairy herds now appear to be the chief clinically significant reservoir for human infection. Sheep and cattle may acquire infection by ingesting contaminated silage. Several outbreaks of human infection have been traced to contaminated food. In one instance, raw vegetables presumably were contaminated on a dairy farm. In another instance, raw milk, ingested as Mexican-type cheese, appears to have been the source. Pasteurized milk may have been implicated in a third outbreak.

According to estimates, the carriage rate of listerial organisms in the gastrointestinal tract of humans approaches 5 percent. Genital colonization has been reported in both men and women; however, this has not been associated consistently with spontaneous wastage. The circumstances under which *L. monocytogenes* becomes an invasive pathogen rather than a saprophyte among either animals or humans currently is not well understood.

DIAGNOSIS

Mother

Listeriosis in pregnancy may present as a minimally symptomatic, nonspecific infectious process (Table 18-1). Mothers may experience a flu-like illness with upper respiratory complaints, fever, and nausea, all presumably related to a transient septicemia. Although mothers may occasionally have signs of severe systemic illness, more often they are asymptomatic. In the latter case, the diagnosis is unsuspected and no treatment is rendered. Within several days, a chorio-

Table 18-1. Diagnosis of *Listeria* Infections

Mother	Child
Clinical	
Often asymptomatic Occasionally "flu" syndrome Rarely, diffuse sepsis	Diffuse sepsis (early onset) Meningitis (late onset)
Laboratory	
Isolation of small gram-positive rods (not diphtheroids) Cultural identification using selective media—specific Cultural confirmation by animal inoculation—limited Serologic documentation by serial titers—limited	Amniocentesis or lumbar puncture

amnionitis develops and spontaneous labor ensues. Under these clinical circumstances, congenital listerial infection develops resulting in septic abortion, stillbirth, or a seriously infected baby. Mothers may then continue as asymptomatic genital carriers for several weeks following delivery.

Mothers of infants who develop neonatal sepsis are more often symptomatic than mothers of children who develop late infection characterized by meningitis. Typically, early-onset or congenital listeriosis presents as acute chorioamnionitis characterized by the abrupt onset of fever, uterine irritability, leukocytosis, and fetal distress that is often associated with meconium staining.

Laboratory diagnosis of maternal genital and neonatal listeriosis depends on isolation of the organism from tissue or body fluid by bacterial culture. Sheep blood or tryptose agar are suitable media for growth of *L. monocytogenes*. Since this organism is morphologically similar to a group of ubiquitous organisms collectively called *diphtheroids, L. monocytogenes* may be mistaken for skin contaminants and disregarded. On the other hand, the presence of a heavy growth of gram-positive pleomorphic rods with rounded ends from body fluids that are normally free of bacterial organisms (such as amniotic or cerebrospinal fluid) should prompt suspicion.

Serologic testing is not widely available in the United States; however, it is of value in the diagnosis and epidemiologic surveillance of human listerial disease. Agglutination titers may be detectable during acute infection; however, they rapidly return to normal following clinical recovery and, thus, may not retrospectively confirm infection. Complement fixation testing, if available, has proved useful in supporting the diagnosis, but false-negative titers may occur in culture-documented cases, especially when there is neurologic involvement.

Child

Like group B streptococcal sepsis, neonatal listeriosis has been divided into two serologically and clinically distinct entities. Early-onset listeriosis, frequently associated with serovarities Ia and IVb,

Table 18-2. Treatment of *Listeria* Infections*

Drug	Mother	Child
Ampicillin[a]	100 mg/kg/day	200–250 mg/kg/day
Erythromycin[a,b]	25 mg/kg/day	40–50 mg/kg/day

*Administer drugs intravenously in 4–6 divided doses. (See also Questions and Answers, below, for treatment of asymptomatic colonization with *Listeria*.)
[a]Consider adjunctive use of an aminoglycoside for empiric therapy, pending cultures.
[b]For patients with history of penicillin allergy.

is a diffuse neonatal septic process with pulmonic, hepatic, and neurologic impairment. Characteristically, affected infants are premature and suffer congenital pneumonia associated with rash and hepatosplenomegaly. Neonatal mortality among those infants who are not stillborn is high, approaching 90 percent. This early-onset syndrome of premature birth, in association with congenital infection frequently resulting in stillbirth or severe neonatal sepsis, constitutes granulomatosis infantseptica.

Late neonatal listeriosis, invariably meningitis, has been associated with serovariety IVb in the United States. Characteristically, affected infants are born at term to asymptomatic mothers who retrospectively are demonstrated to be genital carriers of *L. monocytogenes*. Several days to several weeks following birth, these babies develop meningitis. Morbidity and mortality from this illness continue to remain high, even in recent reports. Forty percent of infants with late onset of listeriosis die. Hydrocephalus or mental retardation are frequent sequelae among the survivors.

PROGNOSIS IF UNTREATED

In the preantibiotic era, mortality among newborn infants suffering listerial infections ranged from 50 to 90 percent. Early diagnosis and initiation of therapy continues to be extremely important in determining the ultimate prognosis for neonatal infection. Recent reports of cases in which the diagnosis of neonatal infection was delayed have been associated with case fatality rates ranging from 25 to 50 percent. Among survivors, some cases of serious long-term central nervous system morbidity have ensued.

MANAGEMENT

Listeriosis is seldom a serious disease among healthy, noncompromised adults. The prognosis for the fetus, however, is best if the diagnosis of congenital infection can be established relatively early in the evolution of infection and aggressive parenteral antibiotic therapy can be instituted. Several accounts of timely diagnosis by amniocentesis in clinically suspicious cases have established the diagnosis by Gram's stain of amniotic fluid, revealing numerous leukocytes and gram-positive coccobacilli. Although the organism is frequently sensitive to chloramphenicol or tetracycline, neither is suitable in neonates due to adverse affects of these drugs in children (Table 18-2). Streptomycin has been used, but some resistance to this drug has been reported. Ampicillin has been the drug of choice for maternal or neonatal infection. Erythromycin may be used in instances of penicillin allergy. In general, clinical experience dictates that antibiotic sensitivity testing should be an essential adjunct for good management.

Often, empiric antibiotic treatment for unexplained chorioamnionitis constitutes the initial therapy for this disease. Under such circumstances, the combination of ampicillin and an aminoglycoside consistently provides good antimicrobial therapy. Treatment should be continued for 7 to 10 days when maternal or neonatal infection has been demonstrated. If central nervous system involvement has occurred, therapy should be extended for at least one week beyond the resolution of symptoms.

PREVENTION

The presence of asymptomatic maternal gastrointestinal and genital carriage makes perinatal listeriosis an inevitable possibility in most obstetric patient populations. The circumstances under which such bacteria, when acquired from animal reservoirs, become clinically significant pathogens are not understood. Similarly, perinatal transmission and the circumstances dictating whether ensuing infections are mild or severe are also unknown. Although much has been learned about the possibility of epidemics arising from dairy-herd reservoirs, the sporadic nature with which such events occur makes large-scale preventative strategies difficult to implement at present.

QUESTIONS AND ANSWERS

1. *Listeria is isolated from the cervical culture of an asymptomatic, penicillin-allergic woman with a history of repeated abortions. What therapy is appropriate?*

   Listeria has frequently been implicated as a cause of recurrent abortion in nonhuman animal species. Occasional cases of recurrent abortion in humans have been reported as well. There are also reports of male colonization with qualitative abnormalities in human sperm associated with recurrent abortion. Sperm morphology has reverted to normal in association with subsequent successful pregnancies following therapy. Other reports have not confirmed such associations.

   Erythromycin or tetracycline 25 mg/kg orally in four divided doses per day for two weeks is appropriate therapy for both sexual partners before attempting another pregnancy. Repeat culture should then be obtained. The presence of listeria is not evidence of cause for recurrent abortion, however, and treatment of genital colonization is not a substitute for evaluating other potential causes of recurrent pregnancy loss.

SELECTED READINGS

Barresi, J. *Listeria monocytogenes:* A cause of premature labor and neonatal sepsis. *Am. J. Obstet. Gynecol.* 136:410–411, 1980.

Barza, M. Listeriosis in milk. *N. Engl. J. Med.* 312:438–440, 1985.

Evans, J., et al. Perinatal listeriosis: Report of an outbreak. *Pediatr. Infect. Dis.* 4:237–241, 1985.

Fleming, A., et al. Successful treatment of maternal septicemia due to *Listeria monocytogenes* at 26 week's gestation. *Obstet. Gynecol.* 66:52s–53s, 1985.

Fleming, D., et al. Pasteurized milk as a vehicle of infection in an outbreak of listeriosis. *N. Engl. J. Med.* 312:404–407, 1985.

Halliday, H., and Hirata, T. Perinatal listeriosis—A review of twelve patients. *Am. J. Obstet. Gynecol.* 133:405–410, 1979.

Koh, K., Cole, T., and Orkin, A. Listeria amnionitis as a cause of fetal distress. *Am. J. Obstet. Gynecol.* 236:261–263, 1980.

Larsson, S., Chronberg, S., and Winblad, S. Listeriosis during pregnancy and neonatal period in Sweden 1958–1974. *Acta. Paediatr. Scand.* 68:485–493, 1979.

Lennon, D., et al. Epidemic perinatal listeriosis. *Pediat. Infect. Dis.* 3:30–34, 1984.

Petrilli, E., D'Ablaing, G., and Ledger, W. *Listeria monocytogenes* chorioamnionitis: Diagnosis by transabdominal amniocentesis. *Obstet. Gynecol.* 55:5s–8s, 1980.

Schlech, W., et al. Epidemic listeriosis—Evidence for transmission by food. *N. Engl. J. Med.* 308:203–206, 1983.

19

Mycoplasmas

Of the 11 species of *Mycoplasma* that have been isolated from humans, only *Mycoplasma pneumoniae, Mycoplasma hominis*, and *Ureaplasma urealyticum* are known to cause disease. Mycoplasmas lack cell walls and represent the smallest free-living organisms. Pathogenic mycoplasmas have been shown to cause a variety of infections (Table 19-1).

M. pneumoniae infections are common. The most important disease manifestation is pneumonia, which generally involves both lower lobes but may have any distribution on chest x-rays. Associated problems may include severe hemolytic anemia, vomiting, diarrhea, otitis media, and a variety of rashes. When disease due to *M. pneumoniae* is suspected, cold agglutinins may be measured. The test is positive in 50 to 90 percent of cases, but it may also be positive in about 20 percent of patients with adenovirus pneumonia. The higher the cold agglutinin titer, however, the greater the probability that the infection is due to *M. pneumoniae*. Specific antibodies against this organism can be measured by a variety of techniques including enzyme-linked immunosorbent assay (ELISA), complement fixation, immunofluorescence, or radioimmunoassay. With proper media and experienced personnel, mycoplasmas can be grown in culture, but growth is very slow.

M. hominis is usually found in the genital tract of adults, but may also be isolated from the oral cavity of as many as 5 percent of individuals. In addition to puerperal endometritis and the disease associations listed in Table 19-1, pregnant women colonized by *M. hominis* have been reported in some studies to be more likely to deliver low birth weight infants, but this association is weak. In newborns, *M. hominis* has been occasionally incriminated in the etiology of meningitis, brain abscess, submandibular lymphadenitis, supraclavicular abscess, scalp abscess, conjunctivitis, pericardial effusion, interstitial pneumonia, and urinary tract infections. *M. hominis* grows on blood agar in nonhemolytic pinpoint colonies. On mycoplasma agar, the colonies have the typical "fried-egg" appearance.

U. urealyticum (previously designated T-strain mycoplasma) is frequently isolated from the genital tract. It can be recovered from about 80 percent of sexually active female adolescents, and from 20% of those not sexually active. Among apparently healthy male adults, urogenital tract colonization varies from 7 to 63 percent (mean, 34%). Neonates become colonized during passage through a birth canal infected with ureaplasmas. About one-third of newborn females, and a smaller proportion of male neonates, are colonized with *U. urealyticum*. Colonization sites in newborns include the nose, throat, genitourinary tract, urine, and umbilicus. Colonization tends to decrease after infancy. Because of the relatively high frequency of ureaplasma colonization, it is frequently difficult to establish an etiologic role for these organisms when isolated from clinical material.

U. urealyticum has been associated with a number of conditions as summarized in Table 19-1. An estimated 20 to 30 percent of nongonococcal urethritis cases are caused by this organism. The association of *U. urealyticum* with low birth weight is based on the observation that colonized neonates have significantly lower birth weights

Table 19-1. Mycoplasma-Associated Human Infections

Organism	Stength of Association	Condition
Mycoplasma pneumoniae	Strong	Pneumonia
	Moderate	Bronchiolitis, pharyngitis, upper respiratory infection, myocarditis, pericarditis, encephalitis
Mycoplasma hominis	Strong	Pyelonephritis, pelvic inflammatory disease, postabortal and postpartum fever
	Moderate	Prostatitis, vaginitis, cervicitis
	Weak	Bartholin gland abscess, low birth weight infant
Ureaplasma urealyticum	Strong	Nongonococcal urethritis, prostatitis, urethral syndrome
	Moderate	Epididymitis, involuntary infertility, spontaneous abortion, stillbirth, chorioamnionitis, low birth weight infant, neonatal pneumonia, asymptomatic bacteriuria, urinary tract infection
	Weak	Pelvic inflammatory disease, pyelonephritis

than noncolonized infants, and that low birth weight infants as a group are significantly more likely to be colonized with *U. urealyticum* than larger neonates. Some studies, however, fail to show such an association. Ureaplasmas are twice as likely to be isolated from newborns whose placentas show histologic evidence of chorioamnionitis than from those with normal placental tissues.

Although nonpregnant adults with *Mycoplasma* infections are best treated with tetracycline, this drug should not be used during pregnancy because of its adverse effects on fetal bone development and tooth staining. Instead, erythromycin (500 mg every 6 to 8 hours) should be used for *M. pneumoniae* or *U. urealyticum,* while *M. hominis* can be treated with clindamycin (150 mg to 300 mg every 6 hours).

SELECTED READINGS

Cassell, G., and Cole, B. Mycoplasmas as agents of human disease. *N. Engl. J. Med.* 304:80–89, 1981.

Cherry, J. Mycoplasma and ureaplasma infections. In R. Feigin and J. Cherry (Eds.), *Textbook of Pediatric Infectious Diseases,* 2d ed., p. 1896. Philadelphia: W.B. Saunders, 1987.

Gilbert, G., et al. Bacteriuria due to ureaplasmas and other fastidious organisms during pregnancy: Prevalence and significance. *Pediatr. Infect. Dis.* 5:S239–S243, 1986.

Kass, E., Lin, J., and McCormack, W. Low birth weight and maternal colonization with genital mycoplasmas. *Pediatr. Infect. Dis.* 5:S279–S281, 1986.

Likitnukul, S., et al. Role of genital mycoplasmas in young infants with suspected sepsis. *J. Pediatr.* 109:971–974, 1986.

20 Chlamydia Infections

Chlamydiae are bacteria that live and grow within host cells. Although chlamydia have both DNA and RNA and are surrounded by a cell wall, they lack the enzymes necessary for oxidative phosphorylation; therefore, they are obligate intracellular parasites for at least a portion of their life cycle. Within the genus *Chlamydia,* there are two species: *C. psittaci* and *C. trachomatis*. The former causes psittacosis, a febrile respiratory tract illness resembling viral or mycoplasmal pneumonia. The latter can cause ophthalmic and genitourinary infections in adults and conjunctivitis, pneumonitis, otitis, and gastroenteritis in newborns.

FREQUENCY

Genitourinary infections caused by *C. trachomatis* are now recognized to be the most common sexually transmitted disease in the United States. It has been estimated that 4 million cases occur annually, making chlamydial infections more common in the United States than the estimated number of new cases of gonorrhea, syphilis, and Herpes simplex infection combined. Among certain high-risk patient populations, cervical carriage rates during pregnancy may approach 15 to 20 percent.

Genitourinary chlamydial infections are most prevalent in young, promiscuous, indigent patient populations. Unmarried women, especially those with multiple sex partners who use either no contraception or a nonbarrier method, appear to be at high risk. Epidemiologic studies in the United States, Western Europe, Great Britain, Scandinavia, and the Philippines all suggest that sexually active adolescents using oral contraceptives carry a 15 to 20 percent risk of infection. Women with other sexually transmitted diseases also constitute a high-risk group. Women with symptomatic infection and positive endocervical cultures for gonorrhea, for example, have a 26 to 33 percent incidence of simultaneous chlamydial infection. Thus, women who are concomitantly infected with or who have a prior history of other sexually transmitted diseases should be considered at significant risk for chlamydial infection.

Psittacosis is an uncommon respiratory infection complicating pregnancy in the United States. The disease is usually acquired through contact with infected birds. Although parrots were originally identified as the animal reservoir of disease, poultry and other nonpsittacine birds may also be infected. Public health legislation controlling this disease within avian reservoirs has contributed to a general reduction in the frequency with which such infections are encountered in the United States today.

DIAGNOSIS

Mother

Many adult women with genital chlamydial infection are either asymptomatic or minimally symptomatic (Table 20-1). Diagnostic testing in the former group may be prompted by discovery of another sexually transmitted disease. In addition, mucopurulent cervicitis has been associated with a 50 percent incidence of chlamydial infection.

Table 20-1. Diagnosis of *Chlamydia Trachomatis* Infection

Mother	Child
Clinical	
Most are asymptomatic	Some are asymptomatic
Many associated with other sexually transmitted diseases	Often:
Occasionally:	Conjunctivitis
Premature rupture of membranes	Interstitial pneumonitis
Preterm labor	Otitis media
Chorioamnionitis	Gastroenteritis
Mucopurulent cervicitis	
"Sterile" pyuria	
Laboratory	
Tissue culture isolation from endocervical or urethral cells	Tissue culture isolation from conjunctival, oropharyngeal, genital, or rectal swabs of cells
Direct detection of chlamydial antigen from clinical samples (see Diagnosis, Mother, p. 147)	
Immunofluorescence	
Enzyme-linked immunosorbent assay (ELISA)	

The diagnosis of mucopurulent cervicitis is established by visualization of yellowish mucopurulent endocervical secretions discoloring a white cotton-tipped swab. Ten or more polymorphonuclear leukocytes per high-power microscopic field in a saline suspension of these secretions in the absence of trichomonads establishes the diagnosis. Women with symptoms of urethral irritation and pyuria whose urine specimens show no evidence of infection by Gram's stain or conventional bacteriologic culture are at high risk for chlamydial infection as well. This condition has been designated as the "urethral" or "dysuria-pyuria" syndrome.

Certain serovarieties of *C. trachomatis* cause lymphogranuloma venereum. This sexually transmitted disease presents first as a papule at the inoculation site. Subsequently, ipsilateral lymphadenopathy develops followed by genital edema, ulceration, and scarring as the disease progresses. Draining fistulae and scarring may ultimately develop on the external genitalia. Since the infection spreads through lymph channels, the perineum, rectum, and rectovaginal septum may become scarred, producing significant dystocia and potentially obstructing vaginal birth. Soft tissue dystocia from this process is occasionally sufficient to necessitate cesarean section delivery.

Psittacosis usually presents as a febrile interstitial pneumonitis. The differential diagnosis includes viral or mycoplasmal pneumonia. Since this infection is usually acquired through contact with infected birds, the diagnosis is generally not suspected unless a history of such contact is obtained.

Isolation of *C. trachomatis* from presumptively infected body secretions using tissue culture remains the "gold standard" for definitive laboratory diagnosis. In addition to being somewhat expensive and cumbersome, the tissue culture methodologies that assure reliable recovery are relatively stringent and, consequently, few health care facilities are optimally equipped to perform cultural isolation on a large scale at the present time. Several details are important to enhance the yield of positive isolates if cultural methods are employed. Samples of endocervical or urethral secretions must contain exfoliated (and presumptively infected) cells. Since chlamydia are intracellular parasites, culture of pus alone will be inadequate for successful culture. Swabs used for transport of specimens should not be treated with calcium alginate, which is toxic to chlamydia, nor should they be composed of wood, which may absorb infectious particles. Cotton-tipped, aluminum-shaft swabs are suitable for culture specimens.

Samples should be transported promptly in a sucrose-phosphate buffer solution supplemented with calf serum and antibiotics for rapid inoculation into tissue culture. Delay between obtaining the specimen and beginning tissue culture results in lower yields of positives. Freezing using conventional methods generally reduces the quantity of infective material that can be recovered; consequently, samples should be refrigerated but not frozen if delay in transport to the laboratory is anticipated. In general, tissue culturing methods require 72 to 96 hours for completion. Most laboratories perform a second blind passage step on initially negative specimens to amplify the number of detectable infective particles from initially low-titer positive clinical specimens. Some studies have demonstrated that this second blind passage step will detect an additional 5 to 15 percent of all positives.

Diagnostic methods other than isolation in tissue culture are less sensitive and slightly less specific but are appropriate and may be preferable as cost-effective alternatives in certain patient populations. Although experience with antigen-detection systems applied to directly stained specimens of body secretions has produced variable results compared with tissue culture, some generalizations can be made. Currently, two major rapid direct antigen kits are available commercially. One uses an enzyme-linked immunosorbent assay (immunoperoxidase) and the other, an immunofluorescent indicator system. The sensitivity of either method for endocervical specimens ranges from 70 to 80 percent, and the specificity ranges from 94 to 96 percent. A recent study comparing the immunofluorescent method to tissue culture in a patient population with a 13 percent prevalence of infection noted a predictive value of a positive (PVP) rapid test of only 65 percent. Lower prevalence populations would have even lower PVPs. Of more importance may be the potential 20 to 30 percent incidence of false-negatives from the cervices of asymptomatic individuals subjected to screening. Nevertheless, the cost and labor of tissue culture isolation makes it an impractical albeit scientifically desirable alternative for screening. The rapid direct methods seem most useful for large-scale screening in high prevalence populations.

Papanicolaou smears are not acceptable substitutes for screening or diagnosis of chlamydial infections since their sensitivity ranges from 40 to 60 percent among culture-positive individuals. Serologic testing is of little clinical value since neither seropositives nor seronegatives reliably correlate with infection or absence of infection. The Frei test, a skin test that measures delayed hypersensitivity, is no longer considered a clinically useful diagnostic approach.

Child

Chlamydial infection is the leading cause of conjunctivitis and afebrile interstitial pneumonitis among infants less than 6 months of age in the United States. Recent experience suggests that prior or concomitant chlamydial infection may be associated with a significantly higher prevalence of neonatal otitis media and gastroenteritis in the same childhood population. Although chlamydial infections have not been shown to cause congenital malformation, neonatal infections presumably arise as the result of transfer of infection from mother to baby during parturition. The attack rate among offspring of colonized mothers may be as high as 50 percent. Neonatal chlamydial infections may be asymptomatic at the time of birth, subsequently becoming clinically manifest weeks or even months following delivery.

Several recent reports have raised other clinical concerns regarding neonatal chlamydial infection. A substantial proportion of newborns presenting the chlamydial conjunctivitis treated with topical antibiotic therapy alone subsequently developed chlamydial pneumonitis. Moreover, follow-up studies performed on children seven to eight years after their hospitalization for chlamydial pneumonia of infancy have revealed a significant association with abnormalities of pulmonary function tests and physician-diagnosed asthma among this group of children compared with noninfected controls.

PROGNOSIS IF UNTREATED

Perinatal infections caused by *C. trachomatis* are now recognized as a potentially significant cause of infant morbidity and mortality. Premature amniorrhexis or labor will indirectly contribute to perinatal wastage by resulting in premature birth. Moreover, superimposed neonatal infection, complicating 50 percent of such births, will result in further potential damage if untreated. In some reports, perinatal chlamydial infections have been associated with stillbirth, presumably the result of untreated intrauterine infection. The frequency and circumstances under which stillbirth occurs currently is not understood.

MANAGEMENT

Mother

The treatment of choice for genitourinary chlamydial infections in nonpregnant women is tetracycline. Since tetracycline treatment during pregnancy should be avoided, erythromycin base, 500 mg, or erythromycin ethylsuccinate, 800 mg four times daily for one week, is the preferred treatment for pregnant women (Table 20-2). One recent study reported a cure rate in excess of 90 percent when the ethylsuccinate regimen in four daily 400 mg dosages was employed. Since the neonatal infection rate among offspring of untreated infected women approaches 50 percent, all women in whom chlamydial infection is diagnosed during gestation should receive treatment, cultural follow-up to assure successful eradication of infection, and repeat testing prior to delivery to exclude the possibility of reinfection. The high frequency with which other sexually transmitted diseases are concomitantly present requires that appropriate testing for and treatment of other sexually transmitted diseases should also be initiated.

Child

Many obstetric centers have modified their practices for post-partum ophthalmic prophylaxis as a result of the increasing prevalence of

Table 20-2. Treatment and Follow-up of *Chlamydia Trachomatis* Infection

Mother	Child
Treatment	
Erythromycin base 500 mg qid × 7 days or Erythromycin ethylsuccinate 800 mg qid × 7 days *Avoid* Erythromycin estolate Tetracyclines Treat or culture for other concomitant sexually transmitted diseases	Erythromycin 50 mg/kg/day in divided doses × 14 days
Follow-up	
Repeat cultures 7–14 days following therapy (as test of cure) and prior to delivery (to screen for infection) Perform follow-up serologic test for syphilis and culture for other sexually transmitted diseases, as indicated by initial cultural findings	Cultures as appropriate (test of cure) Culture and treat parents of infected babies

neonatal chlamydial conjunctivitis. Erythromycin ophthalmic prophylaxis, however, has been associated with treatment failures in some infants. Moreover, topical therapy of neonatal chlamydial conjunctivitis is inadequate to prevent subsequent development of infections in other sites (pneumonitis, otitis, gastroenteritis). Since the latter infections may, based on recent experience, convey long-term sequelae, it seems advisable to treat all neonates suffering chlamydial eye infections with courses of oral or parenteral antibiotic therapy. Erythromycin, 50 mg/kg/day for two weeks, appears to be adequate therapy in most cases. Topical antibiotic therapy does not enhance therapeutic response if oral or parenteral treatment is given; thus, the former is no longer considered necessary for the treatment of conjunctivitis. Ophthalmic irrigation with a pH-balanced, buffered ophthalmic solution may be useful adjunctive therapy. An ophthalmologic consultant should assist in the planning and implementation of therapy.

Newborns with chlamydial infections presumably acquire these during parturition; consequently, the parents of such infected babies should be tested and treated for presumptive infection. Since chlamydial infections in newborns may be both delayed in onset and minimally symptomatic following parturition, careful follow-up of all infants at risk should be conducted.

PREVENTION

Since chlamydial infections are the most common sexually transmitted diseases in the United States, screening for selected patient populations during the prenatal period would seem appropriate. In such patient populations, estimates show that noncultural, antigen detection diagnostic systems may be cost-effective if the prevalence of the infection exceeds 10 to 12 percent. In any event, consideration should be given to screening certain high-risk obstetric populations for infection. Pregnant adolescents, women with other venereal diseases, women with histories of substance abuse, and sexual partners of individuals with genitourinary infection should be included in such testing. Following treatment, mothers and infants alike should, ideally, undergo reculture as a test of cure.

QUESTIONS AND ANSWERS

1. *What is the optimal diagnostic test for detecting perinatal chlamydial infections?*

   Although tissue culture isolation provides the greatest accuracy for the diagnosis of chlamydial infections, this approach is not feasible for large-scale testing. Rapid, nontissue culture methods are less cumbersome and expensive but are associated with both false-positive and false-negative test results. In low prevalence populations (10% or less), tissue culture is the diagnostic approach associated with the highest predictive value. On the other hand, unless unequivocal documentation of infection is deemed necessary, treatment based on clinical signs and symptoms may be more cost-effective than either diagnostic approach at the present time. Under all circumstances, the possibility of other, concomitant sexually transmitted diseases should be considered. Diagnosis or treatment for other associated infections as well as cultural follow-up to verify eradication of chlamydial infection are important elements in successful management of such cases.

2. *How should psittacosis that complicates pregnancy be managed?*

   Psittacosis is usually a self-limited pulmonary infection. Oral erythromycin is usually an effective treatment. Erythromycin ethylsuccinate appears to be associated with fewer gastrointestinal side effects when treatment is given during pregnancy compared with other erythromycin alternatives. Erythromycin estolate has been associated with hepatotoxicity during pregnancy and should not be employed for therapy for chlamydial infections. In most instances, neither psittacosis nor erythromycin therapy should have adverse consequences on the fetus. Since pregnancy may alter pulmonary mechanics, women who fail to respond promptly to therapy should be considered at risk for secondary infections and other pulmonary complications. Accordingly, although outpatient therapy may be the initial approach, hospitalization is indicated if a rapid therapeutic response is not forthcoming. Women admitted to the hospital with psittacosis should be placed on respiratory (mask) and contact isolation to prevent exposure of staff and other patients, since spread of psittacosis among humans can occur in a hospital setting.

SELECTED READINGS

Handsfield, H., et al. Criteria for selective screening for *Chlamydia trachomatis* infection in women attending family planning clinics. *J.A.M.A.* 255:1730–1734, 1986.

Lipkin, E., et al. Comparison of monoclonal antibody staining and culture in diagnosing cervical chlamydial infection. *J. Clin. Microbiol.* 23:114–117, 1986.

Martin, D., et al. Prematurity and perinatal mortality in pregnancies complicated by maternal *Chlamydia trachomatis* infections. *J.A.M.A.* 247:1585–1588, 1982.

Sanders, L., Harrison, H., and Washington, A. Treatment of sexually transmitted chlamydial infections. *J.A.M.A.* 255:1750–1756, 1986.

Schachter, J., et al. Prospective study of *Chlamydial trachomatis*. *J.A.M.A.* 255:3374–3377, 1986.

Tipple, M., Beem, M., and Saxon, E. Clinical characteristics of the afebrile pneumonia associated with *Chlamydia trachomatis* infection in infants less than six months of age. *Pediatrics* 63:192–197, 1979.

Weiss, S., Newcomb, R., and Beem, M. Pulmonary assessment of children after chlamydial pneumonia of infancy. *J. Pediatr.* 108:659–664, 1986.

III Parasitic Infections

21

Trichomonas Infections

Trichomonas vaginalis, a flagellated protozoan organism, is the largest of several trichomonads found in humans. A relatively common cause of female genitourinary infection, this organism was first described as a human parasite in the mid-19th century. Only the motile trophozoite form of the organism is associated with genitourinary and perinatal infections. Transmission of this organism from infected mothers to their newborns was first described in 1942.

FREQUENCY

Since trichomonal infections are not considered a reportable disease, their actual incidence is unknown. Recent surveys comparing the prevalence of various infectious vaginitides in certain patient populations suggest that, compared with other infectious causes of vaginitis, trichomonas may be decreasing in incidence. Nevertheless, trichomonal vaginitis remains the third most frequent cause of lower genital tract infection among women. Current estimates attribute 10 to 15 percent of all cases of vaginitis to *T. vaginalis* infection. Although estrogen appears to enhance trichomonal growth in vitro, within defined patient populations, infection appears equally prevalent among both pregnant and nonpregnant women.

In virtually all circumstances, trichomonal vaginitis is a condition encountered in sexually active women. The covariation between the likelihood of infection and level of sexual activity and the association of trichomoniasis with other sexually transmitted diseases lends support to the contention that trichomonal infection is a venereal disease. Occasionally, female newborn infants will acquire infection from their mothers during parturition. Additionally, trichomonads can be recovered from bath water and swimming pools as long as 24 hours following inoculation; however, desiccation or heat rapidly kills them. Thus, the possibility of other, nonvenereal modes of acquiring infection exists, although the likelihood of such routes of transmission is presumably extremely small.

DIAGNOSIS

Mother

Recent studies have suggested that 50 percent of women with trichomonal vaginitis develop an abnormal discharge characterized by foul odor, mucosal irritation, and a moderate amount of yellowish-gray or blood-tinged vaginal discharge. The presence of a nonspecific vaginal discharge or pruritus has not been correlated with a statistically significant incidence of vaginal trichomoniasis. Conversely, a frothy malodorous vaginal discharge is not necessarily pathognomonic of trichomonas infections. Bacterial vaginosis, now considered the most common form of infectious vaginitis, may be associated with this type of presentation, requiring differentiation from trichomonal infection by microscopic examination of the vaginal secretions and, if indicated, further microbiologic studies.

Pelvic examination of women with trichomonal infection often reveals a diffuse inflammation of the genital epithelium. Punctate submucosal patches of hemorrhage may be suggestive of this type of

Table 21-1. Diagnosis of Trichomoniasis

Mother	Child
Clinical	
Asymptomatic	Asymptomatic
Malodorous, discolored discharge	Malodorous discharge
Vulvovaginitis	Urogenital irritation
Dysuria	Irritability
Laboratory	
Saline suspension for trichomonads or white blood cells	Saline suspension for trichomonads or white blood cells
Culture	Culture

infection. Microscopic examination of a saline suspension of vaginal secretions, popularly referred to as a "wet prep," is a useful first step in the diagnostic evaluation of such women (Table 21-1). Under low-power magnification, *T. vaginalis* has a characteristic pear shape with a pointed posterior pole and a more rounded anterior pole from which arise its undulating membrane and a tuft of anterior flagellae. In saline suspensions, these organisms are usually slightly larger than polymorphonuclear leukocytes. Occasionally, trichomonads may exhibit decreased motility, thus necessitating more careful inspection using high dry magnification for diagnosis. The presence of more than 10 leukocytes per high-powered microscopic field regardless of whether trichomonads are visible by microscopy is associated with a statistically higher frequency of trichomonal infection compared with cases when microscopic examination of vaginal secretions reveals fewer than 10 white cells per high-powered field. The presence of white cells under such circumstances differentiates this type of infectious vaginitis from fungal and most bacterial causes. On the other hand, among women at risk on other epidemiologic grounds, the presence of leukocytes in genital secretions should prompt consideration of the possibility of genitourinary chlamydial infection as well. Since other sexually transmitted diseases are associated with trichomonal infection, individuals found to have trichomoniasis should be carefully evaluated for the presence of other venereal diseases as well, regardless of the presence or absence of an inflammatory vaginal exudate.

Papanicolaou smears occasionally suggest the presence of trichomonal infection. Nevertheless, false-positive and false-negative diagnoses may be prompted by cytologic interpretation, and such findings should be confirmed by saline examination of presumptively infected secretions before assuming the diagnosis has been established. In the event that infection is suspected but microscopic examination of vaginal secretions is nondiagnostic, consideration should be given to establishing the diagnosis by cultural isolation. Trichomonads are facultative anaerobes for which cultural methodologies have been greatly simplified and refined. Hollander fluid medium and Diamond's medium may be successfully employed. Microscopic examination of vaginal secretions alone may miss as many as one-half of all women with vaginal trichomoniasis. These women may only be successfully diagnosed by cultural isolation of the organism. Three-fourths of all positive cultures are detectable within 72 hours of sampling, and blind passage of negative cultures increases the yield of positives by an additional 4 percent.

Child

Infants contract *Trichomonas* infection by contact during passage through an infected birth canal. Trichomonads can be found in amniotic fluid after rupture of the membranes, but this presumably occurs as the result of ascending infection from the lower genital tract. The organism appears to be too large for transchorionic spread while the chorioamniotic membranes are intact. There is essentially no evidence implicating trichomonads as a cause of fever during labor. Isolated reports have associated trichomonas with abortion or premature labor; however, a causative relationship has not been proved.

The diagnosis of trichomoniasis in infants may be difficult. Occasionally, vaginal discharge, pyuria, or irritability may prompt the clinical suspicion of infection. The methods of diagnosis in the infant are identical to those employed for the mother.

PROGNOSIS IF UNTREATED

Trichomonas is essentially always a relatively benign, noninvasive inhabitant of the genitourinary tract. Although spontaneous clearing of the parasitic burden may rarely occur, it is unlikely, and resolution of infection generally occurs only with chemotherapy.

MANAGEMENT

All trichomonal infections requiring therapy should be confirmed by wet smear or culture in addition to prompting additional testing for other venereal diseases as appropriate. Metronidazole is the most effective antimicrobial agent for treatment of trichomonal infection (Table 21-2). Although the conventional course of treatment entails administration of 250 mg 3 times daily for 7 days, recent studies have suggested that a single oral dose of 2 g results in equivalent short-term cure. Sex partners of infected women should also receive treatment. Adverse effects associated with metronidazole therapy include a metallic aftertaste, nausea and gastrointestinal upset, and a disulfiram-like intolerance to alcohol if both drugs are concomitantly ingested. The mechanism of action of metronidazole is incompletely understood; however, it appears to disrupt DNA synthesis in susceptible microorganisms. Although infrequent, trichomonal isolates with relative metronidazole resistance have been reported. In general, such infections may be successfully treated by increasing the dose of metronidazole administered. Nevertheless, the most frequent cause of treatment failures is either medical noncompliance by the patient or reinfection from her persistently infected, noncompliant sexual partner. In such settings, single-dose therapy may be a more practical and efficacious approach. Some aerobic and anaerobic bacteria appear to be capable of inactivating metronidazole. If concomitant bacterial infection is suspected, simultaneous treatment of both conditions may be necessary to assure a satisfactory therapeutic response.

Since there appear to be few, if any, permanent sequelae of maternal trichomoniasis, it is difficult to advocate any treatment during pregnancy that encumbers even theoretic risk. Nevertheless, patients occasionally will develop severe symptoms of infection and require

Table 21-2. Treatment and Follow-up of Trichomoniasis

Mother	Child
Treatment	
Local therapy (see Management, on this page) Metronidazole, 2 g, as a single oral dose or Metronidazole, 250 mg PO tid for 7 days Avoid first trimester treatment, if possible Treat consorts	Metronidazole, 10–30 mg/kg in divided doses for 5–8 days
Follow-up	
Evaluate for other sexually transmitted diseases Treat associated bacterial vulvovaginitis Repeat wet smear or culture if symptoms recur	Repeat wet smear or culture if symptoms recur

treatment. As mentioned above, the treatment of choice for trichomoniasis is oral metronidazole. The association of pulmonary, liver, and mammary tumors in rodents with prolonged administration of high doses of this drug has raised concern about its safety. Nevertheless, carcinogenic potential in humans has not been demonstrated. Similarly, theoretic concerns regarding mutogenesis have been raised as a result of bacterial transformation (Ames) tests. At present, the epidemiologic studies available do not substantiate an equivalent risk of mutogenesis in humans. Excessive developmental injury among offspring whose mothers took metronidazole during pregnancy has not been reported, and the drug is not considered to be a teratogen for humans.

Although the risk of fetal malformation or cancer is probably negligible, the perinatal consequences of infection are probably of too little clinical importance to justify the use of this drug in the first trimester unless symptoms are unusually severe. Trichomonal infections pose little if any danger to the pregnancy itself and can be adequately treated with safety later in pregnancy. Occasionally, consideration may be given to topical application of agents such as providone-iodine or clotrimazole once or twice daily for a period of one week. Although such measures may provide short-term relief, they are generally ineffective for long-term cure. Moreover, they will not eradicate organisms from inaccessible areas such as the bladder in cases of trichomonal cystitis. Persistent, symptomatic trichomonal infections during the second and third trimester may prompt consideration of metronidazole therapy and, at the least, should be considered justification for initiating a careful search of other sexually transmitted diseases in the patient and her partner. Infants with symptomatic trichomoniasis or with persistent urogenital trichomonal colonization beyond the fourth week of life can be treated with metronidazole, 10 to 30 mg/kg daily, for 5 to 8 days.

PREVENTION

Prevention of trichomonal infection depends essentially on avoiding contact with infected individuals and treating sexual contacts concurrently with the individuals themselves.

QUESTIONS AND ANSWERS

1. *Is metronidazole therapy for trichomonal infection contraindicated in the breast-feeding mother?*

   Metronidazole rapidly traverses the fetoplacental barrier and is excreted in breast milk. Thus, drug absorption by the breast-feeding neonate probably results in acquisition of therapeutic dosages of drug. Breast milk concentrations of metronidazole following administration of a single 2 g dose to lactating women are substantially reduced 24 hours following the conclusion of therapy. Although metronidazole is not routinely recommended as therapy in nursing mothers, a single 2 g dose for trichomoniasis followed by abstention from breast feeding for 24 hours may represent a reasonably efficacious therapeutic approach that subjects infants to a greatly reduced amount of metronidazole. In most cases, a single 2 g dose given to nursing women should not be harmful to the infant even though it will ingest metronidazole in the milk.

SELECTED READINGS

Beard, C., et al. Lack of evidence for cancer due to use of metronidazole. *N. Engl. J. Med.* 301:519–522, 1979.

Erickson, S., Oppenheim, G., and Smith, G. Metronidazole in breast milk. *Obstet. Gynecol.* 57:48–50, 1981.

Goldman, P. Metronidazole. *N. Engl. J. Med.* 303:212–218, 1980.

Hager, W., et al. Metronidazole for vaginal trichomoniasis: Seven day versus single dose regimens. *J.A.M.A.* 244:219–220, 1980.

McLellan, R., Spence, M., and Brockman, M. The clinical diagnosis of trichomoniasis. *Obstet. Gynecol.* 60:30–34, 1982.

Muller, M., et al. Three metronidazole-resistant strains of trichomonas vaginalis from the United States. *Am. J. Obstet. Gynecol.* 138:808–812, 1980.

Smith, R. Incubation time, second blind passage, and cost considerations in the isolation of trichomonas vaginalis. *J. Clin. Microbiol.* 24:139–140, 1986.

22

Toxoplasmosis

The organism that causes toxoplasmosis, *Toxoplasma gondii,* was first isolated in 1908 from the North African rodent, the gondii. In 1923, Janku in Czechoslovakia first recognized the syndrome of congenital toxoplasmosis, hydrocephaly, microphthalmia, and chorioretinitis. The availability of antibody tests to assist in the diagnosis of acute toxoplasmosis has resulted in an increased awareness of this disease.

FREQUENCY

To estimate the frequency of toxoplasmosis in adults, it is necessary to rely on studies that have measured the incidence of antibodies to *T. gondii* during surveys of large groups. Such studies have shown that approximately one-third of adult women in the United States have *T. gondii* antibodies. As would be expected, there is a correlation between increasing age and the incidence of women who are seropositive. It has been estimated that in the United States the incidence of maternal toxoplasmosis during pregnancy is 0.5 percent. Only women who become acutely infected with *T. gondii* during pregnancy can have a child with congenital toxoplasmosis.

Estimates of the incidence of toxoplasmosis in newborns vary with the end point being measured. Gross damage due to toxoplasmosis was apparent at birth in 10 of 20,000 infants studied in the Collaborative Perinatal Research Study. However, most congenitally infected newborns are known to be asymptomatic. Only about 20 percent of newborns with congenital toxoplasmosis have extensive or advanced enough disease to be clinically recognized at birth. The frequency with which asymptomatic infected newborns develop symptomatic toxoplasmosis later on is unknown.

If toxoplasmosis is acquired by a pregnant woman during the first trimester, the infection is transmitted to the fetus about 15 percent of the time. The rate of congenital acquisition increases to approximately 25 percent in the second trimester, and 60 percent in the third trimester. Manifestations of congenital toxoplasmosis are likely to be more severe when the maternal infection is acquired early in pregnancy rather than during the third trimester. Infections that occur very early in pregnancy may cause fetal death and abortion, while more than 90 percent of fetal infections acquired in the third trimester are asymptomatic.

DIAGNOSIS

Mother

Maternal toxoplasmosis may be asymptomatic, or there may be a mild mononucleosis-like syndrome. Ten to 20 percent of infected mothers may have lymphadenopathy. Posterior cervical lymphadenopathy may be the most frequent clinical finding associated with acute maternal toxoplasmosis. In contrast, when ocular manifestations of toxoplasmosis have been the index finding, the disease is usually chronic rather than acute.

While the organism may be isolated in the research laboratory by inoculating animals with biopsied tissue, serologic tests are used for

Table 22-1. Diagnosis of Acute Toxoplasmosis

Mother	Child
Clinical	
Suspicion of infection based on: Lymphadenopathy Mononucleosis-like symptoms History of raw meat ingestion History of close contact with possibly infected cats	Suspicion of infection based on: Maternal history, clinical disease, or serologic findings Antenatal diagnosis based on: Ultrasound findings, amniotic fluid culture, and umbilical cord blood sampling Clinical findings in symptomatic newborn Any of the following: Chorioretinitis, convulsions, abnormal head size, rash, hepatosplenomegaly, lymphadenopathy, jaundice, fever, pneumonitis
Laboratory	
Serologic testing (seroconversion, significant titer increase, or positive IgM test) ELISA Hemagglutination Indirect immunofluorescence Sabin-Feldman dye test Placental histology	Serologic testing as in mother; IgM test is diagnostic when positive Nonspecific: abnormal CSF, anemia, intracranial calcifications on x-ray, thrombocytopenia

routine clinical diagnosis. Traditionally used serologic tests include the Sabin-Feldman dye test and the indirect fluorescent antibody test (Table 22-1). Hemagglutination tests have been performed also. More recently, enzyme-linked immunosorbent assay (ELISA) methodology has been introduced for serodiagnosis of *Toxoplasma* infections and has become widely used. The diagnosis of acute toxoplasmosis is made by seroconversion from negative to positive, by a significant increase in antibody titer, or by detection of IgM *Toxoplasma* antibodies. Specific IgM antibodies to *Toxoplasma* can be measured by indirect fluorescent antibody or ELISA techniques. The duration of IgM *Toxoplasma* antibody in serum is variable, but usually is less than six months following acute infection.

Prenatal diagnosis of fetal toxoplasmosis may be accomplished by isolation of *T. gondii* from amniotic fluid or by testing umbilical vein blood sampled by sonar-guided transabdominal needle puncture. However, experience with this approach is limited, and no predictive value can be assigned to a negative finding at this time.

If toxoplasmosis has been suspected before delivery, it is useful to examine the placenta histologically for *Toxoplasma* cysts. The placenta should be fixed in formalin and not refrigerated or frozen, to avoid lysis of the organisms and false-negative histology. A positive examination of the placenta after term delivery will support the diagnosis of acute maternal infection during pregnancy and predict neonatal toxoplasmosis for the overwhelming majority of newborns.

Child

The clinical signs of toxoplasmosis in newborns are characteristic but not specific. Signs of florid congenital toxoplasmosis may include chorioretinitis, convulsions, jaundice, hydrocephaly or microcephaly, fever or hypothermia, hepatosplenomegaly, lymphadenopathy, vomiting, diarrhea, cataracts, microphthalmia, optic atrophy, rash, and pneumonia (Table 22-1). When toxoplasmosis is symptomatic, chorioretinitis is the most common single clinical manifestation found in the newborn period. It may be the only finding present at birth, or it may develop in the first weeks or months of life in an infant who was infected before birth.

Nonspecific laboratory abnormalities seen in symptomatic cases of congenital toxoplasmosis include abnormal cerebrospinal fluid, anemia, abnormal bleeding, and intracranial calcifications. Cerebrospinal fluid findings include xanthochromia, leukocytosis (predominately monocytes), and high protein content.

Whether prompted by clinical signs, laboratory studies, maternal history, or a policy of serologic surveillance, serologic testing remains the best method for diagnosing congenital toxoplasmosis. The fluorescent antibody test and the ELISA test have been modified to measure the concentration of IgM *Toxoplasma* antibodies. Thus, it is possible, under ideal circumstances, to detect both fetal and maternal asymptomatic infections and to discriminate passive transfer of maternal antibodies to the fetus from true fetal infections. While rheumatoid factor (IgM against maternal IgG) produced by the fetus has been shown to cause some IgM tests for *Toxoplasma* antibodies to be falsely positive, such false-positive tests can be eliminated by special treatment of the sera. Although a true positive IgM test establishes the diagnosis of acute toxoplasmosis, the test may be negative in more than 50 percent of infants with definite congenital toxoplasmosis. Newborns infected with *T. gondii* at or near paturition will have antibody-negative cord blood. Clinical manifestations and antibody response will occur during the neonatal period.

MANAGEMENT

Mother

Since the prognosis for the untreated mother is excellent, unless she has impaired defenses against infection, specific treatment is generally unnecessary for maternal recovery. It is not necessary to isolate a pregnant patient who has toxoplasmosis. Although a pregnant woman may transmit the disease to her fetus, it is impossible for her to transmit the disease to anyone else, since the infecting organisms are tissue-bound and not excreted.

The drugs available in the United States for treatment of toxoplasmosis are pyrimethamine and either sulfadiazine or triple sulfonamides. Pyrimethamine has significant potential toxicity as a folic acid antagonist, and could be teratogenic if given during the first trimester. Treatment regimens (Table 22-2) use folinic acid supplements to minimize such toxic effects. It seems that folinic acid protects against bone marrow depression without decreasing the effectiveness of pyrimethamine against *T. gondii*. The sulfa drugs may have unfavorable effects on the fetus by displacing bilirubin and thereby increasing the risk of kernicterus if given just before delivery.

Whether the risk of fetal damage due to intrauterine toxoplasmosis is sufficient to warrant the hazards to the fetus of therapy during the

Table 22-2. Management of Acute Toxoplasmosis (Drug Therapy)

Mother*	Child
Exact regimen for best results has not been established Pyrimethamine 25 mg orally daily + sulfadiazine 1 gm orally qid for 28 days.[a-d] Concurrently give folinic acid 6 mg IM or orally 3 times/week Delete pyrimethamine during 1st trimester Delete sulfadiazine at term Treatment is *not* needed for women with positive serologic test for toxoplasmosis before pregnancy Treatment is *not* needed for maternal recovery from acute infection unless host defense mechanism is compromised Isolation is *not* necessary	Exact regimen for best results has not been established Pyrimethamine 1 mg/kg/day orally for 3–4 days, then 0.5 mg/kg/day for 21–30 days + sulfadiazine 25 mg/kg orally 21–30 days.[a-d] Concurrently give folinic acid 2–6 mg IM or orally 3 times/week. May repeat therapy up to 3 times in first year of life, depending on clinical evidence of disease activity Isolation is *not* necessary Serologic follow-up of asymptomatic antibody-positive infants is recommended at 4–6 week intervals to allow treatment or retreatment. When serologic titer is rising or unchanged, treatment is desirable If titer falls to zero, disease is not present Neuroophthalmologic follow-up is recommended to detect early eye manifestations.

*When diagnosis of acute toxoplasmosis has been made during first 20 weeks of pregnancy, inform patient of possible fetal damage so that abortion may be considered.
[a]Monitor toxicity or therapy with biweekly CBC and platelet count.
[b]If there is evidence of clinically active inflammation, corticosteroids may be given concomitantly with other therapy.
[c]Longer duration of treatment may be needed.
[d]4–5 day half-life of pyrimethamine may require reduction in dosage or increased interval between doses.

first trimester of pregnancy remains uncertain. In some cases, the pregnant woman who has been infected with acute toxoplasmosis during early pregnancy may wish to be aborted, since the risk of having a subsequent pregnancy infected by toxoplasmosis is virtually zero. Treatment with pyrimethamine and sulfadiazine during the second and third trimesters can reduce the incidence of congenital toxoplasmosis, although the degree of effectiveness is uncertain. For patient counseling the efficacy of drug therapy for preventing congenital toxoplasmosis may be estimated at 50 percent. Treatment of the infected mother appears to succeed in preventing fetal infection in part by acting in the time period between maternal infection and transmission to the fetus. If drug therapy for toxoplasmosis is desired during pregnancy the regimen shown in Table 22-2 might be considered.

Spiramycin has been used for toxoplasmosis in France. This drug has not been approved yet for use in the United States. Spiramycin appears to demonstrate minimal transplacental distribution. Apparently it works against *Toxoplasma,* which would otherwise increase on the maternal side of the placenta.

Child

Symptomatic toxoplasmosis in the newborn should be treated without hesitation despite the potential toxicity of the treatment. A treatment program is suggested in Table 22-2. Isolation of infants with toxoplasmosis is unnecessary in the nursery, since organisms are not shed.

The decision to treat for toxoplasmosis becomes more difficult when the diagnosis is suspected but unproved. In cases where there is some evidence of damage, active disease, or a positive IgM antibody test, treatment is justified. When the only evidence of infection is a positive standard serologic test, the IgM-specific test should be obtained from the newborn. Asymptomatic infants with only a positive non-IgM serologic test should usually be observed initially without chemotherapy. In the absence of active infection, the antibody titer due to passive transfer from the mother should decrease at approximately 50 percent per month. At three to four months of age, the presence of antibody produced by the infant can be calculated, as suggested by Remington (1983), and then treatment can be started if indicated.

If cord sera were used for the newborn's first serologic test, which was positive, a second specimen obtained by venipuncture may be useful for an IgM antibody test. This second test would exclude the possibility of a false-positive test result due to contamination of the original specimen by maternal blood. Treatment should be started for infants whose titers rise during serial testing or do not fall.

PREVENTION

Women can acquire toxoplasmosis during pregnancy by eating raw meat containing *T. gondii* cysts, or by ingestion of *T. gondii* oocysts excreted in the feces of infected cats. Thus, in the United States, congenital toxoplasmosis can be substantially decreased by having susceptible women avoid eating meat that has not been thoroughly cooked or thoroughly frozen and by avoiding close contact with infected cats. An acutely infected cat sheds oocysts for only two weeks and is infectious for approximately that period. Toxoplasmosis in cats may be significantly reduced by feeding cats only cooked, canned, or dry food and by preventing the pet from eating wild rodents that may carry the organism. The pregnant woman should also avoid exposure to soil or litter that may contain the infectious feces from cats. Since oocysts in cat feces require incubation to become infectious, additional protection may be achieved by changing the cat litter daily.

It is technically possible to screen for toxoplasmosis antibodies by adding a serologic test for toxoplasmosis to the laboratory work routinely done on all pregnant women while receiving antenatal care, or at the time of delivery. Whether or not a screening program will become a part of routine care depends on estimates of cost and benefit. In areas that have very low rates of congenital toxoplasmosis, falsely positive serologic tests can be expected more often than true positives. Physicians should be alert to the availability of suitable testing facilities in their geographic areas. Testing is currently recommended for patients presumptively exposed for the first time to *T. gondii* during pregnancy.

QUESTIONS AND ANSWERS

1. *What percentage of women are susceptible to toxoplasmosis?*

Serologic surveys of various ethnic and geographic groups have demonstrated that in the United States approximately two-thirds of the adult women lack antibodies to *T. gondii*. The opposite situation seems true in Paris, France, where less than 20 percent of the adult population lacks antibodies to *T. gondii*.

2. *How often during pregnancy should a woman be tested for toxoplasmosis?*

The need for serologic testing depends on (1) the prevalence of toxoplasmosis in the area and (2) the degree of patient or physician concern about risk. Ideally, a patient's *Toxoplasma* antibody status would have been known before she conceives. A woman with antibodies prior to conception is not at risk to deliver a baby with congenital toxoplasmosis.

An ambitious goal would be to attempt to detect asymptomatic toxoplasmosis during pregnancy. Such a program would involve at least a serologic test when the patient first sees her obstetrician, and then a follow-up test to detect either a rising antibody titer or a seroconversion from negative to positive.

If an abortion is being considered, then serologic testing would have to be done early in pregnancy at a time when abortion might be feasible. If the physician would consider treatment during pregnancy, then additional serologic screening for toxoplasmosis could be done late in pregnancy.

3. *If the initial screening serology showed a high titer, what should be done next?*

No definitive answer can be made on one serologic test even if the titer is high. A second specimen should be drawn from the patient and sent to the same laboratory that tested the first specimen. At the same time that the second specimen is tested an aliquot of the first specimen should be tested again. If a high titer is confirmed but there is no further increase in antibody titer, the physician must decide on clinical and epidemiologic findings if the high titer reflects an acute infection during pregnancy. A further two-tube increase in titer would confirm acute infection. Testing for IgM *Toxoplasma* antibody may be useful in discriminating recent from remote exposure. A negative IgM test would indicate that the screening serologic test reflected infection that began more than three weeks before testing. A positive IgM test would support the diagnosis of acute infection.

SELECTED READINGS

Alford, C., Jr., Stagno, S., and Reynolds, D. Congenital toxoplasmosis: Clinical, laboratory and therapeutic considerations, with special reference to subclinical disease. *Bull. N.Y. Acad. Med.* 50:160–181, 1974.

Daffos, F., et al. Prenatal management of 746 pregnancies at risk for congenital toxoplasmosis. *N. Engl. J. Med.* 318:271–275, 1988.

Desmonts, G., and Couvreur, J. Congenital toxoplasmosis: A prospective study of 378 pregnancies. *N. Engl. J. Med.* 290:1110–1116, 1974.

Fuchs, F., Kimball, A., and Kean, B. The management of toxoplasmosis in pregnancy. *Clin. Perinat.* 1:407–422, 1974.

Remington, J., and Desmonts, G. Toxoplasmosis. In J. Remington and J. Klein (Eds.), *Infectious Diseases of the Fetus and Newborn Infant.* Philadelphia: W.B. Saunders, 1983.

Sever, J. Perinatal Infections Affecting the Developing Fetus and Newborn. In H. Eichenwald (Ed.), *The Prevention of Mental Retardation Through Control of Infectious Diseases.* U.S. Public Health Service No. 1692. Washington: U.S. Government Printing Office, 1968.

Teutsch, S., et al. *Toxoplasma gondii* isolated from amniotic fluid. *Obstet. Gynecol.* 55:2S–4S, 1980.

Wilson, C., and Remington, J. What can be done to prevent congenital toxoplasmosis? *Am. J. Obstet. Gynecol.* 138:357–363, 1980.

Wilson, C., et al. Development of adverse sequelae in children born with subclinical *Toxoplasma* infection. *Pediatrics* 66:767–774, 1980.

23

Malaria

Malaria is a relapsing febrile illness caused by four species of the protozoan parasite *Plasmodium*. Naturally occurring infection is transmitted to humans by the bite of *Anopheles* mosquitoes. The fever patterns characteristic of untreated malaria were recognized and described by Hippocrates. Effective chemotherapy became available during the 1600s, when missionaries associated with Spanish explorers in Peru reported the antipyretic properties of an extract of the bark of the cinchona. Later, synthetic antimalarial agents were developed, yet drug resistance and toxicity remain problems for chemoprophylaxis and therapy.

FREQUENCY

Malaria is found worldwide in areas where there are both sufficient numbers of *Anopheles* mosquitoes and infected humans to continue the cycle of disease. Although endemic malaria is no longer a risk in the United States or Europe, the disease is still found in parts of Central America, South America, the Dominican Republic, Haiti, Africa, the Middle East, the Indian subcontinent, Korea, Southeast Asia, and Oceania. The degree of risk within countries in endemic areas is generally greater in low-altitude rural areas in warm weather than in cities.

Travelers returning from endemic areas are a risk group when there has been inadequate malaria prophylaxis while traveling or premature discontinuation of prophylaxis on return. When such persons develop symptomatic malaria, proper diagnosis and management may be delayed. Morbidity and mortality can be substantial in such circumstances. The mortality for untreated first attacks of malaria due to *P. falciparum* in susceptible individuals can be as high as 25 percent. While other species of *Plasmodium* do not usually produce fatal disease, recurrent disease episodes can produce significant debilitation.

It has been generally believed that malaria has a detrimental effect on pregnancy, with an increased incidence of abortions, premature births, and stillbirths associated with symptomatic malaria. Also, the converse has been suggested (i.e., malaria is worsened by pregnancy). It has been suggested that such worsening is in part due to accumulation of the parasites in the placental bed. If the mother has had malaria, plasmodia can be found in the placenta approximately 80 percent of the time. More precise measurement of risk during pregnancy requires more precise measurement of the immune status of the pregnant woman.

At least partial immunity develops during the natural course of untreated malaria. This immunity includes specific IgG antibodies, which serve to protect the fetus from congenital malaria. Epidemiologic studies of congenital malaria have shown the condition to be quite rare among the newborns of mothers native to endemic malarious areas, despite histologically proved placental infestation. This presumed passively transferred protection has been shown to last for several months post partum. While data on the frequency of congenital malaria among babies of nonimmune mothers are scanty, when such a woman has had acute malaria during pregnancy, the incidence of congenital malaria may be as high as 1 to 4 percent.

MECHANISM OF INFECTION

In the cycle of natural malaria infection, humans are the intermediate hosts and *Anopheles* mosquitoes are the definitive hosts. Infection is transmitted from mosquito to man by sporozoites found in the infected mosquito's saliva. The sporozoites enter human liver parenchymal cells, where each sporozoite can develop into thousands of merozoites that rupture out of the liver parenchymal cells to invade red blood cells. As further asexual replication, red blood cell rupture, and invasion of other red blood cells occur, clinical disease is produced.

The usual incubation period from time of mosquito bite until symptomatic human disease develops is approximately 10 to 28 days; however, the incubation period may be extensively prolonged, particularly if the patient was taking chemoprophylaxis at the time of infection. After the first few febrile episodes, the asexual *Plasmodium* replication and red blood cell rupture may become synchronous so that febrile episodes recur at regular intervals. Fever due to *P. vivax* or *P. ovale* infection may recur every other day, while fever due to *P. malariae* may recur every third day. Since replication may remain asynchronous with *P. falciparum* infection, the fever pattern is variable.

Malaria becomes infective from human to mosquito once some of the replicating merozoites have developed into sexual forms called *gametocytes*. The gametocytes can continue the malaria cycle only if ingested by an *Anopheles* mosquito. Within the mosquito, development of the *Plasmodium* requires another 10 to 21 days before disease can be transmitted back to a human. The details of transmission of malaria from mother to fetus remain unclear, but such transmission is apparently favored by maternal parasitemia during labor and delivery.

DIAGNOSIS

Mother

Characteristic clinical manifestations of malaria in adult humans include muscle aching, joint pain, headache, abdominal pain, chills, and fever (Table 23-1). Chills may be as mild as a chilly sensation or as severe as uncontrollable shaking. Temperature elevations during subsequent febrile episodes can be as high as 41° C (106° F).

On physical examination, splenomegaly is a consistent finding. Variable features include hepatomegaly and edema. Particularly severe manifestations of widespread organ involvement can occur with *P. falciparum* infection. The variable array of manifestations may be clinically confusing in any given case. Cerebral manifestations can include delirium, coma, convulsions, and paralysis. Pulmonary manifestations can include coughing and pneumonitis. Gastrointestinal manifestations include vomiting, diarrhea, melena, and persistent pain. In a syndrome of severe *P. falciparum* infection called *blackwater fever*, there is massive hemolysis, hemoglobinuria, and acute renal failure. A grave prognosis has been associated with blood parasite densities greater than 10 percent.

No clinical finding of this protean disease is pathognomonic. The diagnosis of malaria is made by demonstrating the asexual forms of *Plasmodium* on stained specimens of peripheral blood (Table 23-1).

Table 23-1. Diagnosis of Acute Malaria

Mother	Child
History	
Travel in endemic area, or artificial exposure such as narcotics addiction	Acute malaria during pregnancy in nonimmune mother
Clinical	
Common Fever (may show relapsing pattern every 48–72 hr) Headache Nausea and vomiting Hepatosplenomegaly Unusual Diarrhea Cough Dyspnea Delirium Seizures Coma Paralysis Jaundice Acute renal failure	May be asymptomatic at birth, with incubation period up to 30 days before symptoms develop Any of the following may be found: Fever Vomiting, diarrhea, poor feeding Pallor, jaundice Hepatosplenomegaly Acute renal failure Respiratory dysfunction Central nervous sytem dysfunction
Laboratory	
Smear of peripheral blood (*definitive test*) Each species of *Plasmodium* has distinguishing morphology Thin smear—Wright's stain or Giemsa stain Thick smear—Giemsa stain or Field stain Parasite density >10% associated with poor prognosis Hemolytic anemia Hyperbilirubinemia (secondary to hemolysis)	Smear of peripheral blood, as in mother *definitive test* Hemolytic anemia (common) Hyperbilirubinemia secondary to hemolysis Placental histology positive for *Plasmodium* (risk factor only, not definitive for diagnosis in newborn)

While identifying gametocytes establishes the diagnosis of malaria infestation, the asexual forms must be seen to confirm acute infection. An ordinary Wright's stained thin smear may be adequate for initial diagnosis. Subsequently, thick smears stained with Giemsa or other special stains may be used by appropriate experts for identification of the specific species of *Plasmodium* that is present.

Child

The baby may be affected by maternal malaria without acquiring the disease itself. Severe malaria may be associated with abortion, fetal demise, or stillbirth. Lower than expected birth weight has been demonstrated among babies born to mothers with positive blood smears for *Plasmodium* in areas where the disease is endemic; however, it remains for further studies to clarify the complex interaction of fever, nutritional changes, prematurity, and fetal growth retardation.

Newborns infected with malaria may be born asymptomatic, but have the diagnosis established by a positive blood smear. Although diagnosis of maternal malaria may have been made separately and the placenta may demonstrate many plasmodia, only a minority of such babies at risk will have positive blood smears. Such babies may develop symptomatic illness of varying severity from 8 to 30 days of age. In most cases, passive transfer of maternal antibodies provides some protection.

Clinical manifestations of congenital malaria include hepatosplenomegaly, anemia, jaundice, decreased renal function, fever, poor feeding, vomiting, diarrhea, and a variety of neurologic changes. Specific diagnosis depends, as in the adult, on identification of asexual forms of *Plasmodium* in blood smears.

MANAGEMENT

Mother

When acute malaria has been diagnosed, chloroquine is the drug of choice for all species except resistant strains of *P. falciparum* (Table 23-2). Chloroquine may be given orally unless obtundation or vomiting preclude that route. Therapeutic drug levels are easily achieved by intramuscular injection. Alternatively, the severely ill patient can be given intravenous quinine for initial therapy. Chloroquine produces remission of symptoms within 24 to 36 hours by killing the *Plasmodium* in circulating red blood cells. Lack of response within that time is clinical evidence of drug resistance or an erroneous diagnosis.

In the most severe cases, drug therapy alone may be insufficient to prevent death. Exchange transfusion has been reported as a successful and necessary adjunct to chemotherapy for fulminant *P. falciparum* infection when a major proportion of erythrocytes have been parasitized (Kramer et al., 1983). Exchange transfusion might be considered for cases in which the blood parasite density exceeds 10 percent and there is impairment of renal function, cerebral function, or blood coagulation sufficiently extensive to lead to death or severe morbidity if not promptly reversed. Aggressive transfusion management requires access to a hospital adequately equipped for emergencies of this type.

Since *P. vivax* and *P. ovale* persist in exoerythrocytic forms in the liver, symptoms will recur when recurrent rupture of infected liver cells relapses parasites into the blood. Since neither *P. falciparum* nor *P. malariae* persist in the liver, recurrence is not expected after appropriate therapy for the disease; however, reinfection can occur. Thus, it is recommended that chloroquine therapy be continued on a weekly schedule (300 mg base/week) while the patient remains in an endemic area and for six weeks after leaving the area. For patients who remain in an endemic area, the goal of therapy is suppression rather than eradication of infection, based in part on the belief that eradication of all malaria parasites from the body may lead to loss of immunity and increased susceptibility to symptomatic reinfection.

In order to kill the exoerythrocytic forms of *P. vivax* or *P. ovale*, treatment with primaquine is recommended for men and nonpregnant women after the patients have left an endemic area and completed chloroquine therapy. Primaquine is highly active against in-

Table 23-2. Management of Acute Malaria

Mother	Child
P. vivax, P. ovale, P. malariae, and nonresistant *P. falciparum*	*P. vivax, P. ovale, P. malariae,* and nonresistant *P. falciparum*
Severely ill patients Chloroquine 300 mg (base) IM q 6 hr, or quinine 600 mg IV over ≥ 30 min, repeated q 6–8/hr until oral therapy feasible, then chloroquine 300 mg orally q 24 hr for 2 doses	Severely ill newborns Chloroquine, 5 mg/kg IV to start, then repeated in 12–24 hr depending on severity of symptoms
Mildly ill patients Cloroquine (base) 600 mg orally to start, then 300 mg at 6, 24, and 48 hr	Mildly ill newborns Chloroquine, 10 mg/kg orally to start, then 5 mg/kg orally at 6, 24, and 48 hr
Follow-up with chloroquine chemoprophylaxis 300 mg (base) orally each week until patient has been out of endemic area for 6 weeks	Follow-up with chloroquine chemoprophylaxis 37.5 mg (base) total dose orally each week
Primaquine 15 mg (base) orally daily for 14 days (for cure of exoerythrocytic *P. vivax* and *P. ovale*, after pregnancy completed and patient has left endemic area)	
P. falciparum resistant to chloroquine	*P. falciparum* resistant to chloroquine
Severely ill patients Quinine 600 mg IV over 2 to 4 hrs, repeated q 8 hr until oral therapy feasible (max 1800 mg/day), then 650 mg PO tid to complete 10 days therapy plus Pyrimethamine 25 mg bid orally for 3 days plus Sulfadiazine 500 mg qid orally for 5 days	Severely ill newborns Quinine 25 mg/kg/day. Give 1/3 of daily dose IV over 2 to 4 hr; repeat q 8 hr until oral therapy feasible, then 20 to 30 mg/kg/day in 3 divided doses to complete 7–10 days therapy
Mildly ill patients Quinine sulfate 650 mg tid orally for 3 days therapy plus Pyrimethamine and sulfadiazine as above	Mildy ill patients Oral quinine regimen as described above for 7–10 days
Follow-up with chloroquine chemoprophylaxis to suppress *other Plasmodium* species if patient remains in a malarious area, plus Pyrimethamine-sulfadoxine (25 mg pyrimethamine and 500 mg sulfadoxine) orally once weekly. The use of this drug is relatively contraindicated in pregnant women at term and in newborns	
When pyrimethamine is used, toxicity may be minimized by giving folinic acid 6 mg IM or orally 3 times a week	

trahepatic forms of *P. vivax* or *P. ovale*, although it is relatively inactive against the same species in red blood cells. Since primaquine can cause hemolytic anemia when glucose-6-phosphate dehydrogenase (G-6-PD) deficiency is present, the patient's blood should be tested for G-6-PD deficiency before primaquine therapy.

When drug-resistant *P. falciparum* has been diagnosed by either failure of chloroquine or known local prevalence of resistant *Plasmodium*, a combination drug regimen has been recommended. A high cure rate has been achieved by administering quinine, pyrimethamine, and sulfadiazine together (Table 23-2).

Although these drugs each have potential for significant toxicity, the hazard of untreated falciparum malaria in a nonimmune pregnant woman is sufficient to justify their use. The more common toxic effects of quinine include tinnitus, decreased hearing, and decreased vision. Pregnant women with malaria may be more likely to develop hemolytic anemia after quinine therapy than nonpregnant women. Quinine also has been thought by some to be capable of causing abortion, congenital deafness, or congenital blindness; however, these claims have been challenged.

The toxic potential of pyrimethamine is related to its action as a folic acid antagonist. Macrocytic anemia may develop after excessive use. Although pyrimethamine has been shown to be teratogenic for animals, the doses used for treatment of human malaria are so low that teratogenic effect is unlikely. Pyrimethamine toxicity may be minimized by giving folinic acid concurrently. This does not reduce the therapeutic effect of pyrimethamine.

When sulfadiazine or a long-acting sulfonamide is used with pyrimethamine, a synergistic therapeutic effect against *Plasmodium* is achieved. Thus, the combination of the two agents allows a therapeutic effect with reduced toxicity; however, sulfadiazine's potential for enhancing the hazard of neonatal hyperbilirubinemia should be recognized when the drug is given shortly before delivery.

Child

Drug selection for treatment of neonatal malaria is analogous to that appropriate for the mother. Chloroquine is the drug of choice, unless the infecting organism is chloroquine-resistant *P. falciparum*. Then, quinine would be used (Table 23-2).

Malaria in newborns is sufficiently uncommon that there is not a well-defined treatment plan beyond use of chloroquine or quinine. Although it would be a clinical experiment in selected cases of resistant *P. falciparum* infection, pyrimethamine and sulfadiazine might be used concurrently with folinic acid. Maternal and fetal drug toxicity considerations have been reviewed. (See Management, Mother.) In addition, infants are susceptible to chloroquine overdose manifest by cardiovascular collapse. The route of chloroquine treatment should be oral (by gavage if need be) except when there is severe vomiting or cerebral manifestations. Follow-up treatment with primaquine for congenital *P. vivax* or *P. ovale* infection is not needed since there has been no exoerythrocytic (liver) stage of disease.

PREVENTION

In an effort to reduce the worldwide public health hazard of malaria, two strategies have been used: (1) mosquito control and (2) treatment of infected humans. While these measures were successful in eradicating malaria from the United States and Europe, worldwide malaria eradication does not seem feasible in the near future. Mosquitoes have shown an ability to become resistant to contact insecticides, and the insecticides have been a cause of increasing concern as environmental hazards rather than as a shield against disease attack.

Furthermore, *P. falciparum* has shown the capacity to develop resistance to a variety of chemotherapeutic agents. Future progress in malaria control may be enhanced by development of an effective vaccine, but this is still an area of research rather than practical therapeutics.

For individuals at risk, chemoprophylaxis and efforts to minimize exposure to infectious mosquitoes are the mainstays of clinical malaria control. If an individual cannot avoid a malarious area, risk can still be reduced by mechanical and behavioral considerations. *Anopheles* mosquitoes have feeding activity primarily between dusk and dawn. During these hours human risk can be reduced by remaining within well-screened areas, or by wearing long clothing, head coverings, and mosquito repellent when out of doors.

Pregnant women who may be exposed to malaria should take chloroquine chemoprophylaxis on the same weekly schedule as when not pregnant (Table 23-2). For pregnant women who have left malarial areas, chloroquine should be continued for at least six weeks after the last possible exposure. Then, primaquine may be given to prophylactically eliminate any possible exoerythrocytic forms of *P. vivax* or *P. ovale* if it is felt to be clinically appropriate, based on an assessment of the intensity of the previous exposure to malaria. If primaquine is to be used, the patient should be checked first for G-6-PD deficiency. For many women, it is appropriate to defer primaquine until after delivery, provided they are aware of the symptoms of malaria and agree to seek medical assistance promptly if symptoms develop after stopping chloroquine.

There is no satisfactory regimen for chemoprophylaxis against chloroquine-resistant *P. falciparum*, but it has been suggested that amodiaquine (400 mg base orally each week) may be somewhat efficacious. In areas where the likelihood of exposure to chloroquine-resistant strains of *P. falciparum* is high, the use of pyrimethamine-sulfadoxine *in addition to* chloroquine should be considered. The hazards of the medication for a pregnant woman should be balanced against the risk of acute malaria. (See Management, Mother, p. 170). In addition to the risks described earlier, severe cutaneous reactions including erythema multiforme, Stevens-Johnson syndrome and toxic epidermal necrolysis have been reported among travelers taking multiple doses of pyrimethamine-sulfadoxine in addition to chloroquine for prophylaxis. A practical plan for a pregnant traveler with less than three weeks planned exposure might be to carry three pyrimethamine-sulfadoxine tablets to take all at once for empiric therapy should fever occur where no medical help is available. In counseling travelers, it is reasonable to advise pregnant women to avoid any substantial risk of exposure to chloroquine-resistant *P. falciparum* by rearranging itineraries. For babies in areas of malaria risk, chemoprophylaxis is generally not recommended for the first month of life. Newborns of immune mothers may have received some passive protection from transplacental passages of maternal IgG and may receive additional protection via breast milk. Mechanical protection of newborns from mosquito exposure is usually achieved by remaining indoors and judiciously using nets to screen out mosquitoes. As older babies are exposed to possibly infectious mosquitoes, chemoprophylaxis can be achieved by giving chloroquine in liquid form or by attempting to disguise the crushed tablet in food (Table 23-2).

QUESTIONS AND ANSWERS

1. *What precautions are reasonable to prevent iatrogenic spread of malaria from an ill, hospitalized patient?*

   Needle and blood contact precautions are reasonable in areas where no further contact with *Anopheles* mosquitoes is expected.

2. *What management is recommended for a female Foreign Service employee who has left malarial areas but still notes periodic fever, which she treats with leftover chloroquine tablets?*

   Attempt to establish the specific diagnosis of recurrent malaria by blood smear analysis. Rule out other diseases, and then treat as appropriate for diagnosis.

SELECTED READINGS

Centers for Disease Control, U.S. Dept. H.H.S. Congenital malaria in children of refugees—Washington, Massachusetts, Kentucky. *Morbidity and Mortality Weekly Report* 30(5):53–55, 1981.

Centers for Disease Control, U.S. Dept. H.H.S. Recommendations for the prevention of malaria in travelers. *Morbidity and Mortality Weekly Report* 37(17):277–284, 1988.

Drugs for parasitic infections. *Med. Let. Drugs Ther.* 28:9–17, 1986.

Kramer, S., Campbell, C., and Moncrieff, R. Fulminant *Plasmodium falciparum* infection treated with exchange blood transfusion. *J.A.M.A.* 249:244–245, 1983.

Main, E., et al. Treatment of chloroquine-resistant malaria during pregnancy. *J.A.M.A.* 249:3207–3209, 1983.

McGregor, I., et al. Malarial infection of the placenta in the Gambia, West Africa; its incidence and relationship to stillbirth, birthweight, and placental weight. *Trans. R. Soc. Trop. Med. Hyg.* 77:232–244, 1983.

IV

Fungal Infections

24

Candidiasis

Candida albicans, a dimorphic gram-positive yeast, is one of several fungi that exist as normal components of the microflora of human skin and mucous membranes. In the genital mucosa, approximately 80 percent of all fungal organisms present are *C. albicans. Torulopsis glabrata* constitutes an additional 15 percent of the fungal flora. Occasionally, other species of *Candida,* such as *C. tropicalis* and *C. parapsilosis,* may also be encountered. These latter organisms may present special problems with regard to persistent vulvovaginal infection. Thrush, the oropharyngeal infection of neonates born through birth canals infected with *Candida* spp., was first described in the 1940s.

FREQUENCY

Fungal vulvovaginitis, chiefly caused by *C. albicans,* is second only to bacterial vaginosis as the most commonly encountered infection of the vagina. According to estimates, one-third of all pregnant women harbor *Candida* on genital surfaces. Sixty to 90 percent of those who are colonized during pregnancy develop symptoms of vulvovaginal irritation. Moreover, the prevalence of infection increases as gestation progresses. One theoretic explanation for the predilection of pregnant women to develop this infection involves the hormonal influences of pregnancy. Estrogen, especially at the high levels found during pregnancy, enhances the deposition of glycogen in vaginal epithelial cells. This may facilitate candidal growth. Animal studies have demonstrated that estrogen is necessary to make the genital epithelial surface susceptible to colonization by *C. albicans.* Altered carbohydrate tolerance, more likely to develop among women during pregnancy, may also favor fungal growth. Whether pregnancy constitutes a condition in which cell-mediated immunity is altered remains controversial. Recently it has been proposed that some women who suffer recurrent candidal vaginitis may have suppressed immune responsiveness to this organism, thus decreasing their ability to limit fungal proliferation. Whether such factors will ultimately be demonstrated to be clinically important determinants of infection during pregnancy remains to be proved. Nevertheless, the estrogen-mediated facilitation of candidal binding to the vaginal mucous membrane and the presence of cytosol receptors for estrogen on *Candida* that facilitate germination both strongly support the hypothesis that pregnancy favors fungal growth.

Systemic candidiasis is a relatively rare event among obstetric and neonatal populations, occasionally occurring without apparent predisposing cause. On the other hand, women whose pregnancies are complicated by other significant debilitating conditions (such as sepsis and superinfection, renal failure, or immunosuppressed states) occasionally develop systemic candidal infection as a complication. In general, candidal vulvovaginitis is a much more common local infection.

DIAGNOSIS

Mother

Vulvovaginal candidiasis characteristically produces intense discomfort. The chief symptom is pruritus; however, occasionally a sensation

Table 24-1. Diagnosis of Candidiasis

Mother	Child
Clinical	
Asymptomatic Vulvovaginitis Pruritus Dysuria Dyspareunia Curd-like discharge	Congenital infections Systemic sepsis Meningitis Pneumonia Cutaneous lesions with skin eruption Superficial neonatal infections Thrush Perianal rash
Laboratory	
Culture Potassium hydroxide wet smear for hyphae and yeast forms	Culture

of vaginal burning may also be present (Table 24-1). Dysuria and dyspareunia may result from the associated mucositis. A white flocculent discharge, especially in association with intense vaginal mucosal erythema, is highly suggestive of fungal infection. The classic white, "cottage cheese" particulate discharge often found to be adherent to the vaginal sidewalls is not invariably present, however, when monilial vaginitis occurs. When an inflammatory vaginal mucosal reaction is present, there may be extensive vulvar excoriation from scratching. Occasionally, such mucosal lesions may be mistaken for herpetic ulceration.

A presumptive diagnosis of infection caused by *C. albicans* may be made by microscopically examining vaginal secretions for hyphae and yeast forms. Microscopic inspection can be facilitated by suspending the vaginal secretions in a 10 percent potassium hydroxide solution. The visualization of pseudohyphae establishes the diagnosis. On the other hand, absence of microscopic evidence of infection does not exclude this possibility, since 30 to 50 percent of women with subsequently culture-verified infection fail to show evidence of fungus at the time of microscopic examination of vaginal secretions. In clinically suspicious cases where the microscopic examination is negative, the diagnosis may be confirmed by fungal culture. Nickerson's or Sabouraud's media are especially useful for fungal isolation. Exfoliative cytology is notoriously unreliable as a diagnostic tool. Fewer than one-half of all cases of fungal vulvovaginitis are diagnosed by Pap smear.

Child

Oropharyngeal candidiasis of the neonate (thrush) is a common pediatric problem. Colonization of the newborn's alimentary tract occurs during passage through the birth canal. The attack rate in offspring of vaginal carriers has been estimated to be as high as 50 percent.

Although quite rare, true congenital candidiasis of the fetus has been reported. Such infections usually result in disseminated sepsis

Table 24-2. Treatment and Follow-up of Candidiasis

Mother	Child
Treatment	
Topical antifungal therapy Polyenes 100,000 U bid for 2–3 weeks Imidazoles 100–200 mg for 7–10 days Povidone iodine gel/douche for 1–2 weeks Gentian violet USP 1% in weekly topical applications	Congenital (systemic) candidiasis Amphotericin B Superficial neonatal infections Oral nystatin, 1–2 ml of 100,000 U/ml suspension qid for 10 days
Follow-up	
If symptoms persist, reevaluate (see Prevention, p. 190)	Individualize dosage and duration of therapy If symptoms persist, reevaluate in two weeks

with hemorrhage and necrosis of the heart, lungs, and other vital organs. Isolated case reports of candidal meningitis, pneumonia, and septicemia have also been reported, occasionally associated with the presence of a foreign body in the mother's genital tract (such as an intrauterine device or surgical suture). Although retrospective study of such cases suggests that the majority arise as a result of ascending infection from the lower maternal genital tract following occult amniorrhexis, there is some evidence to suggest that invasion of intact chorioamniotic membranes may be possible.

PROGNOSIS IF UNTREATED

Candidal vulvovaginitis and neonatal oral candidiasis are variably symptomatic. It is possible for either infection to exist in a relatively less pathogenic and more saprophytic state for arbitrarily long periods of time, requiring no therapy unless symptoms develop. In contrast, congenital candidiasis is rarely asymptomatic and, thus, virtually always prompts treatment.

MANAGEMENT

Topical antifungal therapy is usually adequate treatment for vulvovaginal candidiasis during pregnancy (Table 24-2). Currently available families of drugs appropriate for therapy during pregnancy include the imidazoles (miconazole and clotrimazole) and the polyenes (nystatin). These agents may be used in either ointment or suppository form. Recent studies have demonstrated that use of vaginal tablets rather than ointments is associated with less loss of the therapeutic agent as a result of vaginal leakage. This may also explain why many women prefer using vaginal tablets or suppositories rather than topical creams. During pregnancy, recurrences are likely unless extended courses of treatment are administered. Consequently, dosages of imidazoles ranging from 100–200 mg/day for a minimum of seven days should be utilized. Twice daily applications of nystatin,

100,000 units, should be prescribed for two to three weeks. There is no evidence that systemic treatment using other antifungals decreases the frequency with which recurrent fungal infections occur during pregnancy. Moreover, the theoretical concerns associated with risk of maternal toxicity and unknown teratogenic consequences preclude unqualified use of systemic antifungals until more information about their consequences for pregnancy become available. Other topical therapies such as povidone iodine and gentian violet have been advocated as fungicides, but are occasionally irritating to the genital mucous membranes themselves and may stain undergarments unless care is taken.

Thrush is treated with oral nystatin, 400,000–600,000 units/day in four divided doses. Vulvovaginal and perianal infections may be concomitantly treated using topical nystatin cream. Congenital systemic candidiasis requires the use of systemic antifungal agents such as amphotericin B under close pediatric or medical supervision.

PREVENTION

Little can be done to prevent candidal vulvovaginitis during pregnancy. Although rectal and vaginal strains of fungus frequently appear to be identical within the same individual, treatment of gastrointestinal reservoirs has failed to consistently decrease the frequency of recurrent infection. Presently, the gastrointestinal tract should be regarded as a potential source of reinfection. Since oral nystatin therapy probably has little perinatal consequence, it may be considered as an adjunctive therapy when persistent or severe recurrent infections complicate pregnancy. Fungal vulvovaginitis is occasionally sexually transmitted, and treatment of an associated candidal balanitis should be considered in instances of recurrent vulvovaginal disease. Uncircumcised men may harbor subclinical infections under the foreskin. Eighty percent of women whose sexual partners have candidal infection are themselves infected with the identical fungal serotype. Nevertheless, no scientific evidence has substantiated the contention that treatment of men will decrease the recurrence rate among women with recurrent monilial infections.

Conditions that may predispose to fungal overgrowth, such as prolonged use of antibiotics, poor diabetic control, or prolonged administration of steroids, should be avoided when possible. Use of cotton undergarments and skirts rather than nonventilating clothing might minimize intertriginous moisture, thus preventing circumstances that might otherwise promote growth of the organism.

Thrush may be prevented by treatment of infected mothers before delivery; however, more than one-half of those women whose children develop thrush are asymptomatic and, thus, never receive treatment. Other mothers have been treated and symptomatically improve, but fail to clear the infection and receive no microbiologic follow-up.

QUESTIONS AND ANSWERS

1. *What steps are appropriate in evaluating pregnant women with recurrent candidal vulvovaginitis?*

   Almost one-half of all women treated for candidiasis during pregnancy require a second course of therapy. Most, however, are free of the fungus following completion of the second treatment. In instances of recurrent infection confirmed by persistence of symptoms and a positive culture, consideration should be given to treatment of sexual partners and simultaneous treatment of the gastrointestinal reservoir. As mentioned earlier, such approaches have not been demonstrated to be efficacious in preventing recurrences based on limited clinical study at the present time. Nevertheless, the risks associated with such approaches are so minimal that a therapeutic trial should be considered. If oral nystatin therapy is initiated, 2–3 million units in divided doses should be administered for 10–14 days.

Other possible explanations for recurrent infections should also be considered. Occasionally, glucose intolerance during pregnancy is associated with recurrent fungal infections. Until euglycemia is restored, control of these associated fungal infections is extremely difficult. Some species of candida (*C. tropicalis*) are notoriously resistant to conventional antifungal therapies. Since these organisms lack ergosterol, their cell membranes are substantially less responsive to conventional therapy with polyenes and imidazoles.

2. *Are there fetal risks associated with topical antifungals administered during pregnancy?*

   Currently available studies suggest that topical therapy with imidazoles (clotrimazole or miconazole) are more effective than polyenes for the treatment of vulvovaginal fungal infection. The former agents are absorbed in extremely small quantities with less than 1 percent of the total administered dose appearing in the maternal circulation. The consequences of maternal absorption for the fetus appear to be negligible.

SELECTED READINGS

Abrams, L., and Weintraub, H. Disposition of radioactivity following intravaginal administration of ^{3}H-miconazole nitrate. *Am. J. Obstet. Gynecol.* 147:970–971, 1983.

Droegemueller, W., et al. Three-day treatment with butoconazole nitrate for vulvovaginal candidiasis. *Obstet. Gynecol.* 64:530–534, 1984.

Horowitz, B., Edelstein, S., and Lippman, L. *Candida tropicalis* vulvovaginitis. *Obstet. Gynecol.* 22:229–232, 1985.

Larsen, B., and Galask, R. Influence of estrogen and normal flora on vaginal candidiasis in the rat. *J. Reprod. Med.* 29:864–868, 1984.

Levin, S., Zaidel, L., and Bernstein, D. Intrauterine infection of fetal brain by candida. *Am. J. Obstet. Gynecol.* 130:597–599, 1978.

Mamlok, R., et al. A case of intrauterine pulmonary candidiasis. *Pediatr. Infect. Dis.* 4:692–694, 1985.

Milstrom, I., and Forssman, L. Repeated candidiasis: Reinfection or recrudescence? A review. *Am. J. Obstet. Gynecol.* 152:956–959, 1985.

Sobel, J. Epidemiology and pathogenesis of recurrent vulvovaginal candidiasis. *Am. J. Obstet. Gynecol.* 152:924–935, 1985.

25

Coccidioidomycosis

Coccidioides immitis, a dimorphic saprophytic fungus that causes coccidioidomycosis, is an infection endemic in the southwestern United States, northern Mexico, and portions of South America. More than 85 percent of all Americans living in the Southwest demonstrate a reactive skin test for coccidioidin, substantiating the fact that infection is common in this part of the United States. *C. immitis* is found in the soil of endemic areas. In its mycelial form, this fungus releases arthrospores which become aerosolized and infect susceptible individuals who inhale them. Although the majority of individuals who become infected remain relatively asymptomatic, approximately 40 percent develop a febrile respiratory illness. This disease, referred to as *Valley fever, San Joaquin fever,* or one of more than 15 other names, usually results in a mild, self-limited disease that clears spontaneously without treatment.

Possibly owing to subtle alterations in immunologic responsiveness, there appears to be a predilection for coccidioidomycosis to become disseminated during pregnancy. The likelihood of dissemination increases with gestational age. Disseminated coccidioidomycosis is a potentially lethal disease. Anergy to the skin test for coccidioidin may be associated with dissemination. Although fatal disseminated coccidioidomycosis had been described previously, it was not until 1949 that the disease was identified as a potential cause of maternal mortality in areas adjoining the San Joaquin valley in southern California.

FREQUENCY

In addition to southern California, coccidioidomycosis is endemic in southern Nevada, Utah, Arizona, New Mexico, and western Texas. Other countries in the Western Hemisphere have reported high incidences of infection as well, including Mexico, Honduras, Venezuela, Bolivia, Paraguay, and Argentina. Although virtually all inhabitants of endemic areas ultimately develop infection, less than 1 percent of nonpregnant individuals develop disseminated infections. Although the exact frequency of dissemination among pregnant women who become acutely infected is unknown, some series estimate a 20 percent incidence. Pregnant and nonpregnant individuals alike are at substantial risk for mortality when coccidioidomycosis disseminates, especially if meningeal involvement occurs. Dissemination appears to be more likely in non-Caucasian individuals.

DIAGNOSIS

Mother

Following a 7 to 16 day incubation period, an influenza-like syndrome ensues among those who develop symptoms (Table 25-1). Substernal or pleuritic pain is common, occurring in 75 to 80 percent of those developing symptoms. Cough and a low-grade fever are common. Pulmonary findings include lower lobe involvement, frequently with hilar or paratracheal adenopathy. A proportion of individuals acutely infected develop allergic reactions with hypersensitivity. These appear more commonly in women (25%) compared with an overall fre-

Table 25-1. Diagnosis of Maternal Coccidioidomycosis

Nondisseminated (Primary)	Disseminated
Clinical	
Low-grade fever (up to 101° F) Most are asymptomatic Influenza syndrome (40%) Erythema nodosum, erythema multiforme, 5–25%	High fever Clinical or radiologic evidence of extrapulmonary disease (e.g., skin lesions, meningitis, osteoarthritis)
Laboratory	
Positive skin test Increased sedimentation rate Leukocytosis and eosinophilia X-ray shows hilar adenopathy, consolidation, occasionally cavitation or effusion Positive complement fixation test Positive precipitin test	Positive or negative skin test Increased sedimentation rate Leukocytosis and eosinophilia X-ray shows miliary spread, paratracheal adenopathy Rising complement fixation titer (1:64) Isolation of spherules from extrapulmonary sites (e.g., placenta, bone, skin)

quency of 5 percent among all cases. Erythema multiforme, erythema nodosum, conjunctivitis, and arthralgias are all manifestations of such hypersensitivity phenomena, occurring 3 to 21 days after the primary infection and lasting several weeks. The arthralgias associated with coccidioidomycosis have been referred to as "desert rheumatism" by natives of endemic areas.

Dissemination during pregnancy may be associated with a variety of complications. Granulomas can be widespread, occurring in the lung, skin, central nervous system, lymph nodes, bones, and joints. Arthritis, meningitis, and miliary pneumonitis are the most dramatic manifestations.

Laboratory findings include characteristic roentgenographic, hematologic, and serologic findings. Chest x-rays may reveal perihilar adenopathy, lobar consolidation, pleural effusions, and (late in the evolution of disease) pulmonary cavitation. Leukocytosis with occasional eosinophilia and elevation of the erythrocyte sedimentation rate frequently develop. Active or progressive infection is usually associated with a 4-fold elevation in the complement fixation antibody titer. Complement fixation titers greater than 1:32 may be associated with incipient disseminated disease. The coccidioidin or spherulin test is a measure of delayed hypersensitivity like a tuberculin skin test. Although this test is usually positive in infected individuals, those who develop disseminated disease may become anergic and nonreactive.

The clinical presentation, in association with characteristic x-ray and serologic findings, is usually sufficient to establish the diagnosis. Alternative diagnostic approaches may be indicated in special cases. *C. immitis* may be isolated in culture from appropriate clinical specimens such as discharge from skin lesions, sputum, or cerebrospinal fluid. Such isolations have been considered somewhat tedious, requiring pretreatment of specimens with antibiotics before plating on Sabouraud glucose agar. Intraperitoneal inoculation of mice with infected clinical material produces an experimental peritonitis from which the isolation of infectious spherules filled with endospores is diagnostic. Alternatively, pleural biopsies of infected tissues produce characteristic findings of tissue necrosis, frequently with a granulomatous infiltrate caused by fungal invasion. In tissue, infective organisms are double-walled spherules, 30 to 60 microns in diameter.

Child

Although still debated by some, it appears that transplacental spread of coccidioidomycosis does not occur, presumably due to the comparatively large size of infective particles. Reports of presumed congenital infection have recently been reinterpreted as acute neonatal infections acquired by the newborn at parturition by aspiration of infected decidua. The large size of the endospore of *C. immitis* as well as the intense thrombosis of capillaries in the bed of infected placentas argues against transplacental acquisition of infant disease. If congenital infections do occur, they are undoubtedly extremely rare. Perinatal mortality associated with disseminated maternal disease is 50 percent. These deaths are due to fetal immaturity and deaths of undelivered mothers; there is no increase in perinatal deaths among infants born at term.

PROGNOSIS IF UNTREATED

Primary coccidioidomycosis in pregnant and nonpregnant patients alike tends to be a benign, self-limited disease that runs its course and resolves without any definitive therapy, carrying a uniformly good prognosis. Those who recover develop relatively permanent immunity from reinfection.

Disseminated coccidioidomycosis, although rare, is frequently fatal if not treated. Prior to the advent of chemotherapy, 50 percent of individuals with disseminated infection died. Even with chemotherapy, the prognosis for those who develop meningitis remains guarded. Whether impaired cell-mediated immune responsiveness during pregnancy contributes to the apparent increased virulence of coccidioidomycosis remains unresolved. Although other systemic fungal infections have been reported during pregnancy, coccidioidomycosis has been reported more frequently and appears more virulent than other fungal infections.

MANAGEMENT

Primary, nondisseminated coccidioidomycosis in pregnancy requires only symptomatic care (Table 25-2). Termination of pregnancy is not indicated in such patients, since the incidence of disseminated infection, though more common in pregnancy, is still infrequent. "Prophylactic" chemotherapy in nondisseminated cases is not justified. On the other hand, prior to the availability of antifungal treatment, 90 percent of all third-trimester coccidioidomycosis resulted in disseminated infection, and 90 percent of these women died. At present, most experts advocate withholding therapy unless evidence of disseminated infection ensues; under such circumstances, aggressive chemotherapy should be instituted.

Dissemination in pregnancy is heralded by persistent symptoms, worsening chest roentgenograms, rising complement fixation titers, loss of delayed hypersensitivity by skin testing, or evidence of ex-

Table 25-2. Treatment and Prognosis of Maternal Coccidioidomycosis*

Undisseminated (Primary)	Disseminated
Treatment	
Symptomatic, supportive	Symptomatic, supportive
Bed rest	Bed rest
Isolation unnecessary	Isolation unnecessary
Termination of pregnancy not indicated	Termination of pregnancy not indicated
Chemotherapy not indicated	
Follow closely for evidence of dissemination, repeating serologic titers every 2 weeks	Amphotericin B 0.25–1 mg/kg/day IV[a] Recommended maximal daily dose, 50 mg/day[a] Recommended maximal total dose, 1–2 g[a]
Prognosis	
Excellent	50% fatal without chemotherapy Meningitis associated with poorer prognosis, despite chemotherapy

*Data clearly documenting fetal coccidioidomycosis are not available.
[a]See Management, p. 184, for details.

trapulmonic spread of the disease, especially to the meninges. In any of these cases, parenteral treatment with amphotericin B is indicated. Amphotericin B is a polyene antimycotic. This drug binds to cell membrane sterols (specifically, ergosterol) producing leakage of cellular constituents and ultimate lysis and death of fungal cells. At low doses, amphotericin B is fungistatic. At higher doses, it is fungicidal. Therapeutic dosages usually correspond to serum levels of 1 to 2 μg/ml. Drug dosages of 0.5 to 1 mg/kg/day are associated with blood levels in this therapeutic range. There has been much debate regarding the administration of amphotericin B; however, the usual initial approach is to administer 1 to 5 mg intravenously over 2 to 6 hours on the first day. The quantity of drug administered is then doubled each day until a maintenance dose has been reached. In vitro antimycotic susceptibility testing is notoriously unreliable in predicting the clinical response. Nephrotoxic side effects can occur; however, since the drug is not excreted in the urine, decreased renal function does not alter serum levels of the drug. Consequently, the dosage of drug administered should not be reduced in individuals with decreased renal function.

Common side effects of amphotericin B treatment include chills and rigors. Approximately 25 percent of treated individuals develop hypokalemia. During therapy, erythropoiesis is diminished resulting in a normochromic normocytic anemia. Virtually all patients undergoing therapy demonstrate a 40 percent reduction in glomerular filtration rate. Nephropathy can occur, but usually not before 5 g of drug have been administered. Renal damage can be avoided if therapy is stopped once the BUN exceeds 50 mg/dl or the serum creatinine exceeds 3.5 mg/dl. Parenteral administration of corticosteroids can ameliorate drug-associated side effects such as chills and fever. Most patients require continuous therapy for 6 to 12 weeks. During this time, those monitoring treatment should carefully assess therapeutic response and observe for drug-associated side effects.

Amphotericin B crosses the fetoplacental barrier. Some clinical accounts have reported cord blood arterial levels of drug similar to those found in maternal serum at the time of delivery. The fetal consequences of amphotericin B therapy during pregnancy are unknown. No adverse effects have been reported among the infants of the few women who have been treated. Since the fungus is tissue-bound and, thus, not infectious, patients need not be isolated during therapy.

PREVENTION

Little can be done to prevent primary infections in endemic areas. Pregnant women registering in such areas should be screened with a coccidioidin skin test, and pulmonary symptoms during pregnancy should prompt evaluation with chest roentgenography and appropriate serologic testing. Women with primary coccidioidomycosis in pregnancy must be observed closely for evidence of dissemination and treated vigorously if it is suspected. Sporadic reports occur of primary infections due to contact with fomites (cotton or wool exported from an endemic area) and from entry of spores through skin abrasions. Nevertheless, the overwhelming majority of infections occur from inhalation of spores while traveling through or residing in an endemic area, especially during dry months of the year. Avoiding contact with potentially infected dust in such environments may lower the incidence of primary infection in nonimmune susceptible individuals by as much as 50 percent.

QUESTIONS AND ANSWERS

1. *How is a coccidioidin or spherulin skin test performed?*

   Inject 0.1 ml of coccidioidin intradermally. A second intradermal test should be administered simultaneously as an anergic control (mumps antigen, streptokinase–streptodornase, or trichophyton). An area of induration ≥ 5 mm in diameter at 48–72 hours following administration indicates previous antigenic exposure. Evidence of delayed hypersensitivity responsiveness is evidence of immunity to reinfection unless the individual (1) becomes immunologically compromised, or (2) is concurrently suffering from ongoing coccidioidomycosis.

2. *A pregnant woman in the second trimester in an area endemic for coccidioidomycosis develops pulmonary symptoms. The coccidioidin skin test is positive, and the chest roentgenogram is nondiagnostic. How should this patient be treated?*

   This patient should be evaluated promptly with serial serologic testing for ongoing infection. A precipitin test is available and is positive only in recent infections. Rising complement fixation titers with clinical evidence of dissemination mandate therapy. Loss of delayed skin test reactivity is an ominous immunologic sign.

SELECTED READINGS

Harris, R. Coccidioidomycosis complicating pregnancy. *Obstet Gynecol.* 28:401–405, 1966.

Harrison, H. Fatal maternal coccidioidomycosis—A case report and review of sixteen cases from the literature. *Am. J. Obstet. Gynecol.* 75:813–820, 1958.

McCoy, N., Ellenberg, J., and Killim, A. Coccidioidomycosis complicating pregnancy. *Am. J. Obstet. Gynecol.* 137:139–140, 1980.

McGregor, J., Kleinschmidt-De Masters, B., and Ogle, J. Meningoencephalitis caused by *Histoplasma capsulatum* complicating pregnancy. *Am. J. Obstet. Gynecol.,* 154:925–931, 1986.

Medoff, G., and Kobayashi, G. Strategies and the treatment of systemic fungal infections. *N. Engl. J. Med.* 302:145–155, 1980.

Parker, P., and Adcock, L. Pelvic coccidioidomycosis. *Obstet. Gynecol. Surv.* 36:225–229, 1981.

Spark, R. Does transplacental spread of coccidioidomycosis occur? *Arch. Pathol. Lab. Med.* 105:347–350, 1981.

Watts, E., Gard, P., and Tuthill, S. First reported case of intrauterine transmission of blastomycosis. *Pediatr. Infect. Dis.* 2:308–310, 1983.

Index

Index

Handbook of Perinatal Infections

John L. Sever, M.D., Ph.D.
John W. Larsen, Jr., M.D.
John H. Grossman III, M.D., Ph.D.

"...the Handbook is an ideal and handy reference...."
—*The New England Journal of Medicine*
(about the first edition)

This practical handbook draws on the authors' expertise and experience in the fields of infectious diseases, obstetrics, and gynecology to present a clinically oriented review of perinatal infections. Now in a second edition, it offers up-to-date, directly applicable information on the diagnosis and treatment of infections commonly encountered in pregnant women and newborn infants.

Divided into four parts, **Handbook of Perinatal Infections, Second Edition,** offers current information on commonly encountered viral, bacterial, parasitic, and fungal [illegible]

- A historical or epidemiological overview of the infection
- Clinical and laboratory methods of diagnosis in mothers and infants
- Techniques for management and prevention of perinatal infections
- A useful question-and-answer summary of common problems
- Tables summarizing diagnosis and management of major diseases
- Selected readings for further study

Revised and updated for its second edition, the Handbook now includes important new material on AIDS, condylomata acuminata, and chlamydial infections, as well as on parvoviruses.

Illustrated with photographs and line drawings, **Handbook of Perinatal Infections, Second Edition,** is a convenient and authoritative resource for students, residents, and practitioners in the office, in the laboratory, or at the bedside.

Little, Brown and Company